Membrane Transformations in Neoplasia

MIAMI WINTER SYMPOSIA

*Published by North-Holland Publishing Company, Amsterdam, The Netherlands.

MIAMI WINTER SYMPOSIA - VOLUME 8

Membrane Transformations in Neoplasia

edited by
Julius Schultz
Ronald E. Block

THE PAPANICOLAOU CANCER RESEARCH INSTITUTE
MIAMI, FLORIDA

*Proceedings of the Miami Winter Symposia, January 17-18, 1974,
organized by The Papanicolaou Cancer Research Institute, Miami, Florida*

ACADEMIC PRESS   New York and London 1974
A Subsidiary of Harcourt Brace Jovanovich, Publishers

ACADEMIC PRESS, INC.
111 Fifth Avenue, New York, New York 10003

United Kingdom Edition published by
ACADEMIC PRESS, INC. (LONDON) LTD.
24/28 Oval Road, London NW1

Library of Congress Cataloging in Publication Data
Main entry under title:

Membrane transformations in neoplasia.

    (Miami winter symposia, v. 8)
    1.   Cancer cells–Congresses.   2.   Cell membranes–
Congresses.   I.   Schultz, Julius, Date   ed.
II.   Block, Ronald E., ed.   III.   Papanicolaou Cancer
Research Institute.   IV.   Series.   [DNLM: 1.   Cell
transformation, Neoplastic–Congresses.   W3MI202 v. 8
1974 / QZ206 M533 1974]
RC261.M52   616.9'94'07   74-8601
ISBN 0–12–632760–2

CONTENTS

CONTENTS

CONTENTS

SPEAKERS, CHAIRMEN, AND DISCUSSANTS

C. **Abell**, University of Texas, Galveston, Texas

M. Z. Atassi, Wayne State University, Detroit, Michigan

R. Bernacki, Roswell Park Memorial Institute, Buffalo, New York

M. W. Bitensky, Yale University School of Medicine, New Haven, Connecticut

R. E. Block, Papanicolaou Cancer Research Institute, Miami, Florida

Z. Brada, Papanicolaou Cancer Research Institute, Miami, Florida

H. Brandt, University of Miami School of Medicine, Miami, Florida

S. Chatterjee, Michigan State University, East Lansing, Michigan

L. DeLuca, National Institutes of Health, Bethesda, Maryland

H. Eagle (Session Chairman), Albert Einstein College of Medicine, Bronx, New York

B. F. Erlanger, Columbia University, New York, New York

P. H. Fishman, National Institutes of Health, Bethesda, Maryland

I. Fritz, University of Toronto, Ontario, Canada

C. G. Gahmberg, University of Washington, Seattle, Washington

S. Greer, University of Miami School of Medicine, Miami, Florida

L. P. Hager, University of Illinois, Urbana, Illinois

S. Hakomori, University of Washington, Seattle, Washington

H. J. Heineiger, The Jackson Laboratory, Bar Harbor, Maine

H. G. Hempling, Medical University of South Carolina, Charleston, South Carolina

ix

J. Hochstadt, Worcester Foundation for Experimental Biology, Shrewsbury, Massachusetts

V. P. Hollander, Hospital for Joint Diseases, New York, New York

M. Horowitz, New York Medical College, Valhalle, New York

J. Jaroszewski, Naval Medical Research Institute, Bethesda, Maryland

R. W. Jeanloz, Massachusetts General Hospital, Boston, Massachusetts

J. Kallos, Columbia University, New York, New York

G. Koch, Roche Institute of Molecular Biology, Nutley, New Jersey

W. Korytnyk, Roswell Park Memorial Institute, Buffalo, New York

J. Kowal, University Hospitals, Cleveland, Ohio

W. Lands, University of Michigan, Ann Arbor, Michigan

B. B. Lavietes, New York University Medical Center, New York, New York

R. C. Leif, Papanicolaou Cancer Research Institute, Miami, Florida

W. R. Loewenstein (Session Chairman), University of Miami School of Medicine, Miami, Florida

R. Longton, Naval Medical Research Institute, Bethesda, Maryland

M. Lubin, Dartmouth Medical School, Hanover, New Hampshire

W. S. Lynn, Duke Medical Center, Durham, North Carolina

I. MacPherson, Imperial Cancer Research Fund Laboratories, London, England

E. Matthews, Litton Bionetics, Inc., Kensington, Maryland

G. Milo, College of Veterinary Medicine, Columbus, Ohio

M. Morrison, St. Jude Children's Research Hospital, Memphis, Tennessee

K. Muench, University of Miami School of Medicine, Miami, Florida

D. V. K. Murthy, Syntex Research Institute of Biological Sciences, Palo Alto, California

M. Rieber, Center of Microbiology and Cell Biology, Caracas, Venezuela

S. Ristow, University of Minnesota, Minneapolis, Minnesota

R. M. Roberts, University of Florida, Gainsville, Florida

A. H. Romano, University of Connecticut, Storrs, Connecticut

S. Roseman, Johns Hopkins University, Baltimore, Maryland

J. Roth, Biocenter, Basel, Switzerland

H. Rubin, University of California, Berkeley, California

L. Sachs (Session Chairman), Weizmann Institute of Science, Rehovot, Israel

B. Sanford, National Institutes of Health, Bethesda, Maryland

I. Schenkein, New York University Medical Center, New York, New York

J. Schultz, Papanicolaou Cancer Research Institute, Miami, Florida

M. Sherman, Sloan-Kettering Institute, New York, New York

S. Sorof, Institute of Cancer Research, Philadelphia, Pennsylvania

P. A. Srere, Veterans Administration Hospital, Dallas, Texas

S. Steiner, Baylor College of Medicine, Houston, Texas

L. Warren (Session Chairman), University of Pennsylvania School of Medicine, Philadelphia, Pennsylvania

M. J. Weber, University of Illinois, Urbana, Illinois

R. S. Weinstein, Tufts University School of Medicine, Boston, Massachusetts

J. Whitehead, Veterans Administration Hospital, San Francisco, California

J. Wolff, National Institutes of Health, Bethesda, Maryland

PREFACE

Despite the large number of symposia published or unpublished taking place each year, the Miami Winter Symposia has managed to grow in interest. Its purpose has been recognized and its function as a continuing source of knowledge is being fulfilled.

The organizers of the Miami Winter Symposia had in mind to provide an opportunity for communication of new findings in rapidly advancing areas of research. In this way, a forum is presented for the consolidation of the forces of knowledge which provides a possible regrouping of these forces for more definitive focus of attack by those in the field, and a clarification for those who need the knowledge for related problems. For example, within a few months after the disclosure of the discovery of RNA-directed DNA synthesis in 1971, Drs. Temins, Baltimore, Spiegelman, Gallo, and Todaro were presenting their findings at the Miami Winter Symposia, 1972. Dr. Kornberg presented the Lynen Lecture and Dr. Seymour Cohen disclosed new findings in polyamines. "Reverse Transcriptase" was coined shortly before publication of that volume.

Now the seventh volume and its companion, Volume 8, are on cell surfaces. As we go to press, a feature article has appeared in *Science* (183, 1279, 1974) "Biochemistry of Cancer Cells: Focus on the Cell Surface", by J. L. Marx pointing out the major effort in the attack on the cancer problem through the study of cell surfaces. Most of the references in that review are to scientists who participated in the Miami Winter Symposia, 1974.

It is particularly important that both volumes overlap in their coverage more than in the past, reflecting the intense interest in the concern with the cancer problem of investigations in this field.

This volume also constitutes Volume 63 of the I.U.B. Symposium.

ACKNOWLEDGMENTS

Acknowledgment is made here to Eli Lilly, Hoffmann-La Roche, and Smith Kline, and French for their financial contributions. The editors wish also to thank Dr. W. Loewenstein of the University of Miami and Dr. L. Warren of the University of Pennsylvania for suggesting participants for the Symposia. Special recognition is due the girls in the "boiler room" who transcribed the discussions and worked so hard to follow up the edited comments to be included in time for the publication.

Membrane Transformations in Neoplasia

MEMBRANE GLYCOPROTEINS IN NORMAL AND VIRUS-TRANSFORMED CELLS

L. WARREN, J. P. FUHRER, C. A. BUCK and E. F. WALBORG, JR.

Department of Therapeutic Research, School of Medicine University of Pennsylvania, Philadelphia, Pa. 19174 Division of Biology, Kansas State University, Manhattan, Kansas 66502; and University of Texas, M. D. Anderson Hospital and Tumor Institute, Houston, Texas 77025.

The cell surface has been a focus of interest in our attempts to understand malignancy. The surface membrane is undoubtedly involved in such important processes as cell recognition, adhesiveness, lectin binding, virus binding and synthesis, and nutrient transport (1,2). It may play a critical role in the control of cell division. Important antigens reside on the cell surface (3,4). The transformed cell appears to differ from the normal in many of these surface-associated structures and functions and so a host of biochemical studies have been instigated to detect and characterize consistent structural differences between control and malignant cells and their surface membranes.

Glycoproteins are components of membranes, both surface and internal and they are believed to take part in several of the processes described above. It is therefore not unreasonable to see whether significant differences exist between the membrane glycoproteins of normal and malignant or virus-transformed cells. In recent years several workers have made significant contributions to this field.

In general terms, the amount of membrane glycoprotein can change, the extent and character of aggregation may be altered, the location of the glycoprotein within the membrane may be shifted, the polypeptide component of

1

the glycoprotein may be altered and there could be changes
in the carbohydrate moiety. We have been most concerned
with the latter, i.e. alterations of the carbohydrate
component of the glycoproteins of the surface membrane of
cells in tissue culture after transformation.

It is widely believed that the primary chemical
change in the malignant cell is in the nucleic acids. It
is probably a qualitative change. Beyond this we are con-
fronted with the mechanics of the expression of malignancy
and this is what most of the audience at the present
meeting are studying.

I will be describing a difference in the glycoproteins
of control and transformed cells, but the important
question remains unanswered and will remain so for the
present: are the observed differences integral components
of the process of malignancy or, are they merely secondary,
quantitative, casual perturbations? These questions will
be difficult to answer.

We have exploited the double-label method in order to
compare the carbohydrate components of the glycoproteins
of the surface membranes of control and virus-transformed
cells. We grow control cells in roller bottles in the
presence of a ^{14}C-containing carbohydrate precursor (L-
fucose or D-glucosamine) and transformed cells with the
same ^{3}H-containing material. Experiments are occasionally
done with the labels reversed. After the cells have
grown in log phase for 2 or 3 days the cells are washed
and removed from the glass surface with trypsin. The cell
suspension is centrifuged. The supernatant solution,
called the trypsinate, contains material derived from the
superficial layers of the cell--about one quarter of the
cell's L-fucose and sialic acid and about 10% of the cell
protein. The surface membranes are also obtained from the
cells for chromatographic comparison.

The two trypsinates, derived from control and virus-
transformed cells, each labeled with a different isotope,
are mixed and exhaustively digested with pronase so that
glycopeptides bearing only a few amino acids are formed.
These are chromatographed on long columns of Sephadex G-
50 and each tube is counted for ^{3}H and ^{14}C. The surface

membranes isolated from the cells are subjected to the same process (5).

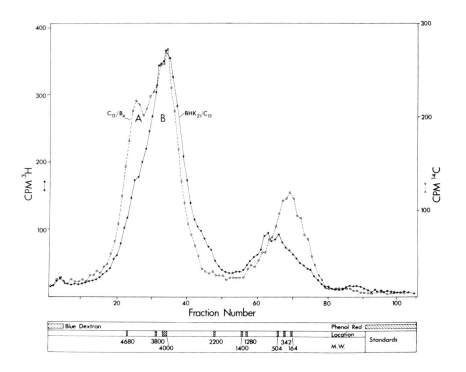

Fig. 1. Double-label elution patterns of pronase digests of trypsinates from a column of Sephadex G50 fine. Material derived from surfaces of BHK_{21}/C_{13} cells (control) and from cells transformed by Rous virus, C_{13}/B_4. The former cells were cultured for 3 days in the presence of ^{14}C-L-fucose and the latter with ^3H-L-fucose prior to trypsinization. Details of method may be found in ref. 5.

In Fig. 1 is seen the results of an experiment in which the trypsinate of the baby hamster kidney cell, BHK_{21}/C_{13} is compared with that of C_{13}/B_4, the same cell transformed by the Bryan strain of Rous sarcoma virus.

3

It can be seen that there is an early-eluting peak of
glycopeptides (peak A) derived from the transformed cell
that is at best only minimally present in the control. It
has a molecular weight of approximately 4600 as shown by
comparison with known standards. The glycopeptides
eluting in the peak B area are smaller, having an approximate molecular weight of 4000.

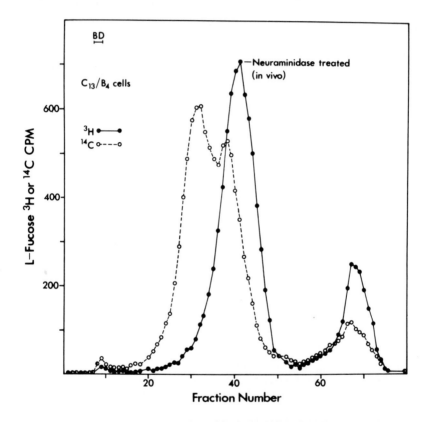

Fig. 2. Elution patterns of surface
glycopeptides derived from C_{13}/B_4 cells
cultured in the presence of ^3H or ^{14}C-L-
fucose. Those cells, labelled with ^3H,
were treated with neuraminidase (V. cholerae) for 1 hour to remove sialic acid
of the cell surface. Both ^3H and ^{14}C-
labelled cells were then treated with

4

trypsin, the trypsinates were mixed,
digested with pronase and chromatographed on a column of Sephadex G50
fine.

It has been shown that the glycopeptides of the peak
A region are larger because they contain extra molecules
of sialic acid, probably two per glycopeptide. If the
glycopeptides are treated with neuraminidase before
chromatography, peak A disappears and the glycopeptides
derived from both kinds of cells cochromatograph. If
living C_{13}/B_4 cells are treated with neuraminidase, then
treated with trypsin to obtain a trypsinate which is mixed
with a trypsinate from C_{13}/B_4 cells not subjected to
neuraminidase the pattern of the pronase digests seen in
Fig. 2 is obtained. The "intact" trypsinate material shows
a peak A & B (dashed line), while the material from the
cells exposed to neuraminidase has lost the A peak (solid
line). In fact the resulting peak has moved to the right
of peak B and is now called peak B'. This shows that the
glycopeptides of peak B also contain sialic acids but in
lesser amounts than do peak A glycopeptides (see below).
The same results have been obtained using neuraminidase
derived from V. cholerae and purified by affinity chromatography (6), C. perfringens, influenza virus and by acid
hydrolysis (0.1 N H_2SO_4, 80°, 1 hr.). It should be emphasized that the control cell, BHK_{21}/C_{13}, also contains peak
A glycopeptides but not nearly as much as does C_{13}/B_4. A
small shoulder or peak is almost always seen in the peak
A region of the elution pattern of material derived from
control cells.

The absence of a prominent peak A in the control cell
pattern could be due to a neuraminidase in this cell which
is absent in the transformed cell. We have looked for
this enzyme in these cells and in the cell medium but
could not find significant amounts of activity; certainly
not enough to account for our results.

The relatively large peak A of transformed cells is
not due to a differential rate of synthesis and turnover
with respect to peak B glycopeptides. Time studies have
shown that the relative sizes of peak A & B remain constant in control and transformed cells no matter what the

5

length of the labeling period. When cells are labeled with isotope for several days, washed and then cultured in non-isotopic medium, the total amount of radioactivity in the cell decreases but the relative size of peak A & B remain constant. Curiously, however, the pronase digests of radioactive glycoproteins of the medium in which control and transformed cells were grown are very poor in peak A glycopeptides. The reason for this is unknown at the present time.

On the other hand, we have found a sialyl transferase which is increased 2.5 to 11 times in the transformed cell that transfers sialic acid (NAN) from its activated form, CMPNAN, to an acceptor, desialylated peak A glyco-peptide derived from the surface of C_{13}/B_4 cells. This may account for the increased levels of peak A glycopep-tides in transformed cells. Before I describe our most recent work on this enzyme I would like to discuss recent observations about the glycopeptides of peak A & B and to summarize information on these structures.

The elution patterns that are seen in Fig. 1 can be obtained using ^{14}C and ^{3}H-L-fucose, D-glucosamine, D-mannose or D-galactose.

It should be emphasized that a peak A is seen not only in transformed cells but in non-transformed controls as a shoulder or small peak. It is however always overshadowed by the relatively large peak A derived from the trans-formed counterpart. The difference we are describing is quantitative.

The formation of peak A glycopeptides appears to be growth-dependent. They are not seen as a peak in materials derived from either control or transformed cells that have become confluent and have essentially stopped dividing. However, if cell division has been arrested in M phase by vinblastine sulfate or at the G1/S interphase with thy-midine, peak A glycopeptides are still formed. It would appear that peak A glycopeptides may be formed when the cell is in any part of the cycle but not when it is in a resting, (G_0) phase while peak B glycopeptides are formed independently.

A prominent peak A is seen in cells derived from a
variety of species (rat, mouse, hamster, chicken) transformed by both DNA & RNA-containing oncogenic virus and in
spontaneously transformed cells. The changes have been
seen in transformed cells of lymphoid, fibroblastic and
epithelioid types (8,9). It is of interest that peak A
of material from 3T3 cells doubly transformed by SV_{40} and
polyoma virus is considerably greater than the peak A
manifested by 3T3 cells transformed by either polyoma
virus or SV_{40} virus alone. 3T3-SV displays only a small
but definite peak A (unpublished).

Peak A is seen in chick embryo fibroblasts transformed by T5, a temperature-sensitive mutant of Rous
sarcoma virus, when grown at a permissive temperature
(36°) where malignancy is expressed but not at a non-
permissive temperature of 40°. (11). Since virus progeny
are produced equally well at both temperatures (10) the
appearance of peak A glycopeptides is not associated with
virus infection per se or virus production. In support
of this statement is the observation that the elution
patterns of glycopeptides derived from chick embryo fibroblasts before and after infection with RAV-1 virus are
essentially identical (11).

Most of our work comparing glycopeptides of control
and transformed cells has been done with trypsinates derived from the intact cell's surface. We have obtained the
same results comparing isolated surface membranes of these
cells. This shows that the glycopeptide patterns are the
same across the entire structure of the surface membrane.
In recent experiments it has been demonstrated that the
relatively large peak A seen in the elution patterns from
surface material is also present in the nuclear (12) inner
and outer mitochondrial and lysosomal membranes as well as
in smooth endoplasmic reticulum (13) (Fig. 3a,b,c).

7

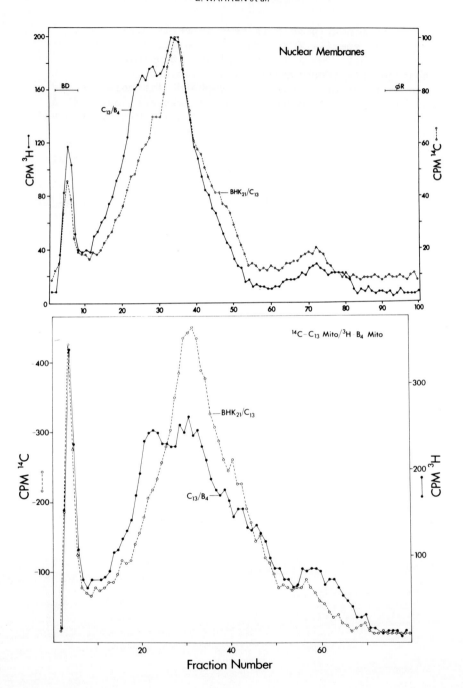

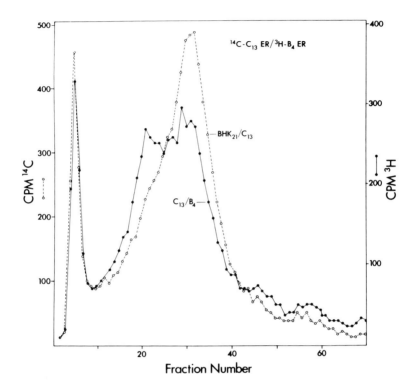

Fig. 3. Double-label elution patterns of glycopeptides derived from various types of membranes of BHK_{21}/C_{13} and C_{13}/B_4 cells. Cells were labelled with ^3H and ^{14}C-L-fucose.

These differences could not have been the result of contamination of inner membrane fractions by surface membrane because cells were treated with neuraminidase before fractionation. As seen in Fig. 2 peak A is eliminated from the surface membrane. If the various isolated internal membranes of control and transformed cells are treated with neuraminidase their chromatographic patterns become the same and peak A disappears. Thus a coordinate change seems to take place in the glycoproteins of the surface and internal membrane systems of the cell upon transformation. If one homogenizes isotopically labeled cells,

digests the entire homogenate and chromatographs on a
column of Sephadex G50 a pattern results that is essentially identical to that seen in Fig. 1.

This rather constant pattern in the membrane glycoproteins suggests that in the addition of carbohydrates
to glycoproteins that are certain, final size modalities
of the carbohydrate moiety, although sugars are probably
added to glycoproteins one by one (14). Some oligosaccharides bound to protein stop accepting sugars during
synthesis when they are of di- or trisaccharide size
(tubes 55 to 80 in Fig. 1). Others stop at about 14
sugars (peak B) others when they contain 16 sugars (peak
A) and still others when they are relatively large,
eluting with blue dextran (Fig. 1). Populations of
protein-bound oligosaccharides of intermediate size are
relatively scarce.

It has been found that if cells are cultured in the
presence of ethidium bromide at concentrations that
reduce growth only slightly, peak A which is barely seen
in the membrane glycoproteins of control cells ($BHK_{21}/$
C_{13}) becomes very prominent and that of the transformed
cell becomes even larger than usual. These changes take
place in the glycoproteins of all the membrane systems of
the cell (15). Ethidium bromide is a phenanthridine dye
that intercalates between bases of DNA especially the
circular forms and also enhances the incorporation of
thymidine into nuclear DNA. Although the effects of
ethidium bromide are multiple and complex it is hoped
that it can in some way be used as a probe in discerning
the relation of the growth-dependent formation of peak A
glycopeptides to nuclear and perhaps mitochondrial events.

We have some information about the location of peak A
& B glycopeptides in glycoproteins. A major aim of our
laboratory is to isolate and purify membrane glycoproteins. We have had some success with columns of
hydroxylapatite (16) and with gel electrophoresis. A
glycoprotein has been obtained which appears to contain
glycopeptides of peak A size alone while others contain
glycopeptides of varying proportions of peak A & B. Thus,
we have tentatively concluded that these glycopeptides
are found in more than one membrane glycoprotein.

In this discussion peak A & peak B have been treated
as entities. In fact, they are each rather complex, consisting of many glycopeptides that are not resolved on
columns of Sephadex G50, Biogel P10 or P30. Further, but
incomplete resolution of these fractions has been obtained
on columns of Dowex-1-acetate and of DEAE Sephadex G25.
We have used high voltage electrophoresis in pyridine
acetate buffer to obtain 3 peaks of material from peak A
after desialylation and 4 peaks from peak B, one of which
is probably a component of peak A since its composition
and sialic acid content is like that of the peak A components and it travels more rapidly, in the peak A area,
in an electrophoretic field. These have been analysed to
get some notion of the differences between peak A & B glycopeptides, although chromatography on columns of G-25
DEAE Sephadex or Dowex-1-acetate clearly shows that they
are not homogeneous. Recently however we have found that
two dimensional chromatography and electrophoresis on thin
layer plates resolves peak A & B materials into a number
of discrete spots that can be visualized with fluoresca-
mine or ninhydrin sprays as well as by autoradiography.
The excellent resolution by this relatively simple and
rapid means should obviate the column procedures.

However, analysis of the subfractions of peaks A
and B of C_{13}/B_4 cells obtained by high voltage electrophoresis on paper reveals a number of interesting points.
(Table 1). The glycopeptides contain, L-fucose, D-glucosamine, D-galactose, D-mannose and sialic acid. The
peak A glycopeptides contain approximately two more
sialic acid and D-galactose residues than do the peak B
glycopeptides but contain one less molecule of D-mannose.
Most of the glycopeptides in peak A contain a molar
equivalent of aspartic acid (asparagine?); those of peak
B contain less. Most contain threonine and serine, as
well as glutamic acid, glycine, and alanine with little
or no valine, isoleucine or leucine. An overall estimate of the molecular weight of peak A glycopeptides is
4300, those of peak B, 3600. The difference is roughly
equivalent to the molecular weight of two sialic acid
molecules.

Repeated attempts to remove carbohydrate from polypeptides by alkaline reduction have failed suggesting

11

TABLE 1

Analysis of subfractions of A and B peaks of C_{13}/B_4 cells

	A1	A2	A3	B1	B2	B3	B4
L-Fucose	1.0	1.0	2.0	1.0	1.0	1.0	2.0
D-Mannose	3.3	4.3	3.5	4.6	4.8	4.9	4.6
D-Galactose	4.8	7.0	5.9	3.1	3.5	4.1	5.8
D-Glucosamine	2.9	3.3	3.6	2.1	3.9	4.1	6.2
Sialic Acid		3.1		0	0.9	1.5	4.5
Asp	0.8	0.7	1.0	0.4	0.3	0.4	1.0
Threo	1.0	0.5	0.6	0.2	0.4	0.3	1.1
Serine	1.3	0.6	0.9	tr	0.1	0.2	0.5
Glut	0.4	0.5	0.9	tr	0.1	0.1	0.7
Glyc	1.5	0.9	1.1	tr	0.1	0.1	0.5
Ala	0.7	0.3	0.4	0.1	0.1	0.1	1.6
Val	0.6	tr	tr	tr	tr	tr	0.4
Isoleuc	0.2	tr	tr	0	tr	tr	tr
Leuc	0.3	tr	tr	tr	tr	tr	0.2
Phenylala	0.8	1.1	0.4	1.0	0.8	1.1	2.0

Carbohydrates were analysed as their alditol acetates by gas liquid chromatography (17), sialic acid by the thiobarbituric acid assay after acid hydrolysis (18). It should be noted that the sialic acid level of unfractionated peak A glycopeptides is given (3.1). Amino acid analyses were kindly performed by Dr. L. Rebhun and Mr. C. Mitchell, Dept. of Biology, University of Virginia.

that the linkages are through a β-glycosylamine structure
involving L-asparagine and N-acetyl-D-glucosamine. L-
fucose is present in all glycopeptides. It is resistant
to the α-fucosidase of C. perfringens despite the fact
that the enzyme is capable of cleaving L-fucose from a
macromolecule, hog gastric mucin. Much of the L-fucose
of both peak A and B glycopeptides, however, is susceptible to purified α-fucosidase of rat epididymus. The
peak B glycopeptides cling to columns of Concanavalin A-
Sepharose while those of peak A pass through.

Finally, I would like to discuss some recent work on
sialyl transferases which appears to be relatively specific for certain types of acceptors and may be responsible
for the synthesis of peak A glycopeptides. Although these
glycopeptides are larger than those found in the peak B
region and probably passed through the peak B size range
during synthesis on a protein, it cannot be assumed that
the precursors of peak A reside in the peak B region,
awaiting to be sialylated. Even the relatively crude,
analytic data suggests several differences between peak A
& B glycopeptides. The sialyl transferase elevated in
transformed cells (7) may only be the last of several
transferases that are increased in amount and are responsible for the appearance of peak A glycopeptides independently of the pathway of peak B glycopeptide synthesis.

In the in vitro sialyltransferase assay with which we
have worked, enzyme is incubated with CMPNAN-^{14}C and
desialylated peak A acceptor, which is obtained from the
surface of C_{13}/B cells. The transferase, if present,
transfers ^{14}C- NAN to the acceptor. The entire incubation mixture is chromatographed on a column of Sephadex
G50. An initial radioactive peak eluting with a blue
dextran marker results from transfer of ^{14}C-NAN to an
endogenous acceptor of unknown character in the enzyme
preparation. A second radioactive peak is a measure of
NAN transfer to added glycopeptide (desialylated peak A
or other glycopeptide). This is followed by an enormous
radioactive peak consisting of unused CMP-NAN-^{14}C (see
Fig. 4). We have studied the kinetic parameters of the
reaction with respect to time, enzyme, CMPNAN, and
acceptor concentrations. The optimum pH is 7.0.

As previously stated the enzyme level is elevated in the transformed cell (C_{13}/B_4, PyY, CEF-SR) but is sharply reduced in amount in both control and transformed cells when they are not dividing and in plateau phase. Further, it is elevated in T5-transformed chick embryo fibroblasts grown at 36° where malignancy is expressed and is reduced to the level found in the control cell at 41° (7). Thus, it is seen that a large peak A and an elevated level of this sialyl transferase go together.

The enzyme appears to have some specificity. While transferase activity, using desialylated peak A as acceptor, is markedly elevated in homogenates of transformed cells over that of controls, transferase activity in the same extracts is approximately the same to the endogenous acceptor in the crude enzyme preparation, to desialylated fetuin and to bovine mucin. Transfer of NAN does not take place to intact peak A glycopeptides (already bearing NAN). It has been found by others that sialyl transferases are generally reduced in transformed cells (19-21) although in another study an elevation in a cell surface transferase has been demonstrated that is probably the same as the one we have described (22).

The enzyme has been found in the surface membrane. Since we now know that peak A glycopeptides exist in the internal membrane systems (13) we are carrying out experiments to see if a sialyl transferase with the characteristics of that found in the surface is also present in these membranes.

Recently we have been collaborating with Dr. Earl F. Walborg, Jr. who, with his colleagues, have isolated a number of glycopeptides from the surface of Novikoff rat hepatoma cells. These glycopeptides cleaved from the cell surface by papain were prepared according to the procedure described by Smith et al (23) and the resolution and nomenclature is the same as the reported for the glycopeptides from rat hepatoma AS-30D. We have desialylated these enzymatically and have tested them as acceptors in our enzyme assay. It can be seen in Table 2 that an homogenate of C_{13}/B_4 cells has 3.5 to 6.7 times more activity than does an homogenate of untransformed BHK_{21}/C_{13} cells. On the other hand, transfer of NAN to endo-

14

genous acceptor in the homogenates is approximately similar.
It should be noted that some glycopeptides are not sialyl
acceptors and in fact seem to inhibit NAN transferase while
in other cases these glycopeptides may actually stimulate
transfer (to endogenous acceptor). This may suggest that
the carbohydrate components of glycoproteins may modulate
transferase activities.

It is of interest that in the experiment described in
Table 2 species boundaries have been crossed in that an
enzyme from hamster cells is transferring NAN to an acceptor derived from rat cells. We tested the possibility
that there might be a human NAN-transferase elevated in
malignancy and capable of transferring NAN to the rat
acceptors. Since cancer cells are probably shedding their
surface membrane (24), the enzyme might be found in human
serum. In Fig. 4 is seen the results of an experiment
where 0.03 ml of normal human serum and the serum of a
woman with a breast cancer were incubated for 40 minutes
with ^{14}C-CMPNAN and desialylated glycopeptide (C-SGP-C) of
rat hepatoma. The incubation mixtures were then chromatographed on a column of Sephadex G-50. It is clear that
activity is dramatically increased in the serum of the
woman with the tumor.

In Fig. 5 is seen the results obtained to date of
testing sera from healthy individuals and those with
various forms of malignancies. Most sera of patients
with malignancies have elevated levels of enzyme. Transfer of NAN to endogenous acceptors was sometimes elevated
in sera of patients with tumors but not to the same extent as transfer to added acceptor. These studies are
continuing and other body fluids are being tested, for
enzyme levels, cerebrospinal fluid, pleural and ascitic
fluids. Further, sera of patients with non-malignant dis-
seases are being tested as controls. We will obtain surface glycopeptides from a variety of human tumors, de-
sialylate them and use them as acceptors. Perhaps the
sensitivity and specificity of the test can be enhanced
by assaying for example serum of a woman suspected of
having a breast carcinoma with acceptor from breast cancer tissue. Whether or nor the sialyl transferase that
we are measuring in human sera is related to the one we
have been studying in homogenates of normal and transfor-

15

Table 2

Added acceptor	Amt(μg)	NAN transferred; cpm/mg protein/hr.					
		Endogenous acceptor		Change	Added acceptor		Change
		BHK_{21}/C_{13}	C_{13}/B_4		BHK_{21}/C_{13}	C_{13}/B_4	
None	0				0	0	
C-SGP	45	4296	5422	1.3	0	0	
C-SGP-A	46	4414	6266	1.4	0	0	
C-SGP-B	50	2222	3112	1.4	2488	16,785	6.7
C-SGP-C	49	2134	3096	1.5	3896	19,556	5.8
DC-1	45	3126	1965	0.6	0	0	
DC-2	45	2666	1644	0.6	2874	9970	3.5
DC-3	45	2118	2296	1.1	1852	9630	5.2
DC-4	45	2726	2933	1.1	4712	22,370	4.8
DC-5	44	3096	2370	0.8	3362	15,674	4.7
C-SGP-A+C-SGP-B		2940			6200		
C-SGP-A+C-SGP-C		3530			6750		

The incubation mixture consisted of buffer, CMPNAN-^{14}C, NAN acceptor and cell homogenate as previously described (7). The resolution and nomenclature of the cell surface glycopeptide acceptor from Novikoff hepatoma cells is the same as that reported for the glycopeptides from hepatoma AS-30D (23).

Incubated for 40 minutes at 37°. Phenol red and blue dextran markers were added and the incubation mixture was chromatographed on a column of Sephadex G-50 fine.

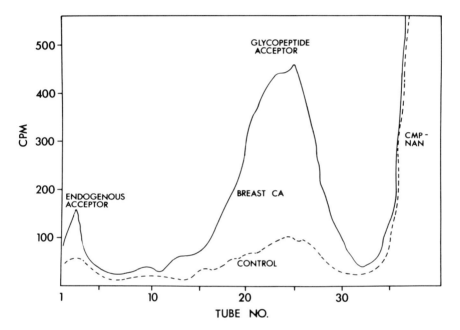

Fig. 4. Assay of sialyl (NAN)-trans-
ferase. Elution pattern of incubation mixture
on a column of Sephadex G50 fine (0.8 X 65 cm).
The incubation mixture consisted of 30 μg of
desialylated glycopeptide acceptor Novikoff
hepatoma C-SGP-C, 10 μg CMPNAN (0.3 μCi),
serum 30 μl and sodium phosphate buffer 0.1
M pH 7.0 containing Triton X 100 & MgCl₂
10 μl. Incubation fo 40 minutes at 37².

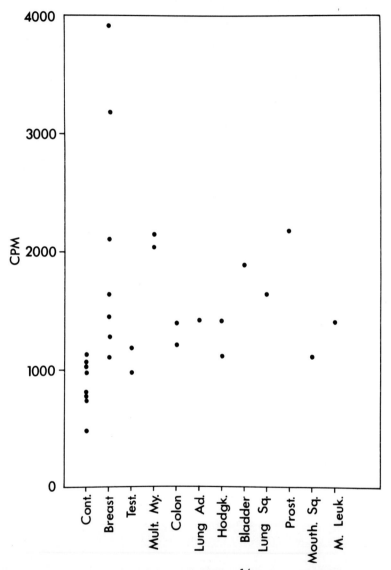

Fig. 5. Transfer of NAN-^{14}C from CMPNAN-^{14}C to glycopeptide acceptor as described in legend of Fig. 4. Sera containing the transferases were obtained through the kindness of of Dr. R. Cooper, Dept. of Medicine (Hematology). Hospital of the University of Pennsylvania.

med cells in culture remains to be determined. If it is, it extends the generality of the change in glycopeptide related to sialic acid described in this and previous papers.

REFERENCES

(1) M. M. Burger in: Current Topics in Cellular Regulation, Vol. 3, eds. B. L. Horecker and E. R. Stadtman (Academic Press, New York, 1971) p. 135; Federation Proc. 32 (1973) 91.

(2) M. Abercrombie and E. J. Ambrose, Cancer Research 22 (1962) 525.

(3) G. Klein, Federation Proc. 28 (1969) 1739.

(4) P. Koldorsky in Handbuch der Allgemeinen Pathologie Vol. 7, part 3, p. 455 (Springer_Verlag, Berlin Heidelberg, New York (1970).

(5) C. A. Buck, M. C. Glick and L. Warren, Biochemistry 9 (1970) 4567; 10 (1971) 2176; Science 172 (1971) 169.

(6) P. Quatrecasas, Biochem. and Biophys. Research Communs. 35 (1969) 531.

(7) L. Warren, J. P. Fuhrer and C. A. Buck, Proc. Nat'l. Acad. Sci. U.S. 69 (1972) 1838; Federation Proc. 32 (1973) 80.

(8) P. Emmelot, Europ. J. Cancer 9 (1973) 319.

(9) W. P. Van Beek, L. A. Smets and P. Emmelot, Cancer Res. 33 (1973) 2913.

(10) G. S. Martin, Nature 227 (1970) 1021.

(11) L. Warren, D. Critchley and I. Macpherson, Nature 235 (1972) 275.

(12) A. A. Keshgegian and M. C. Glick, Biochemistry 12 (1973) 1221.

(13) C. A. Buck, J. P. Fuhrer, G. Soslau and L. Warren, J. Biol. Chem., in press.

(14) S. Roseman in Biochemistry of Glycoproteins and Related Substances, Cystic Fibrosis (Mucoviscidosis) eds. E. Rossi and E. Stoll (Karger, Basel/New York, 1968 p. 244.

(15) G. Soslau, J. P. Fuhrer, M. M. K. Nass and L. Warren J. Biol. Chem., in press.

(16) B. Moss and E. N. Rosenblum, J. Biol. Chem. 247 (1972) 5194.

(17) W. F. Lehnhardt and R. J. Winzler, J. Chromat. 34 (1968) 471.

(18) L. Warren, J. Biol. Chem. 234 (1959) 1971.

(19) F. A. Cumar, R. O. Brady, E. H. Kolodny, V. W. McFarland and P. T. Mora, Proc. Nat'l. Acad. Sci. U.S. 67 (1970) 757.

(20) H. Den, A. M. Schultz, M. Baou and S. Roseman, J. Biol. Chem. 246 (1971) 2721.

(21) W. J. Grimes, Biochemistry 9 (1970) 5083.

(22) H. B. Bosmann, Biochem. Biophys. Research Commun. 49 (1972) 1256.

(23) D. F. Smith, G. Neri and E. F. Walborg, Jr., Biochemistry 12 (1973) 2111.

(24) L. Warren and M. C. Glick, J. Cell Biol. 37 (1968) 729.

This work was supported by grants from the American Cancer Society PRP-28, BC 16C, from the Robt. A. Welch Foundation Grant No. G-354 and the U.S. Public Health Service CA 12526-01 and 1 R01 CA 13992-01. J.P.F. is supported by N.I.H. training grant U.S.P.H.S. 5 T01 AI-00357-05.

The invaluable assistance of Ms. Kerstin Malmstrom and Carol Walz is gratefully acknowledged.

DISCUSSION

I. MacPherson, Imperial Cancer Research Fund Laboratories: You gave evidence that in the RSV (Bryan strain) transformed BHK 21 cell peak A glycopeptide expression and the sialotransferase was minimal in what you called plateau cells. Could you explain what you mean by a plateau in transformed cell cultures?

L. Warren, University of Pennsylvania: If you allow cells, C_{13}/B_4 or BHK 21/C_{13} to divide and then their growth rate flattens off, the C_{13}/B_4 cells divide to a certain point and then they slow up greatly. When they're harvested a few days after they reach not a total but a virtual plateau, the growth rate has a very small slope. If you check then, their enzyme content is low and their peak A is essentially non-existent.

I. MacPherson: Under these conditions the culture would be very acid.

L. Warren: No, no. This was controlled. There was glucose there and the pH was right.

I. Schenkein, N.Y.U. School of Medicine: I don't know whether this is feasible, but could you treat the cell surfaces of living cells with neuraminidase and then from an aliquot show the difference in elution of your peak A, and could you then if you washed the neuraminidase off show resynthesis of this peak A material? Does it come back in other words?

L. Warren: When you remove sialic acid from the surface of a cell you're doing a lot of things. It may be one procedure, but you're knocking sialic acid off of many structures, so you're going to have many consequences. Second of all I would say that in the repair

22

process, after sialic acid is removed, it is not simply a matter of putting sialic acid back. What happens is that turnover will replace the entire sialic acid-bearing protein. The rate of replacement of the sialic acid bearing structure isn't any greater if you do or do not treat with neuraminidase. It's a constant renewal and flushing out and replacement.

I. *Schenkein*: Yes. Okay, thanks.

E. *Matthews, Litton Bionetics*: I was wondering if you took the purified fragments from peak A and treated them with neuraminidase whether you'd generate the same ones that you found in peak B.

L. *Warren*: No, I don't think so. Analysis showed that the peak A glycopeptides differ from the B's although one of the B's looked like an A, I must say these fractionations are most imperfect and I can't come to any categorical conclusions about that.

R. *Bernacki, Roswell Park*: You mentioned that you found peak A glycopeptides in mitochondrial membranes. What was the ratio between the inner and outer membranes?

L. *Warren*: The elution patterns looked quite the same. It's just that there were four times as many counts in the outer membrane as in the inner and I think this agrees with others that the outer mitochondrial membrane is considerably richer in glycoprotein than the inner.

R. *Bernacki*: Also, in your assay for serum sialyltransferase, what were you using as an acceptor?

L. *Warren*: We have used different kinds but mostly Walborg's desialated rat hepatoma glycopeptides, but as I say, we'd like to switch to human glycopeptides derived from various kinds of human tumors.

G. *Milo, Ohio State University*: Dr. Warren, I
have two questions I would like to have you comment on:
1) Is it possible that the ethidium bromide used in
your system at the concentrations you applied to the
cells could possibly act as a mutagen or carcinogen?
The expression of this agent at the cytoplasmic membrane site could be an expression of a phenomenon known
as "transitory malignancy." This transitory phase
could result in shift in glycoprotein synthesis from
normal patterns of synthesis to an altered pattern of
synthesis due to the treatment. The second question, I
would like to have you comment on is: the data you
presented indicating that there is a serum elevation of
sialotransferase activity in patients with breast
cancer may have an alternate interpretation. The
presentation of this data in your last slide was elegantly illustrated. Have you considered that the increase
in sialotransferase activity in the serum could be an
effect of unusual amounts of prolactin or releasing
factors in the serum?

L. *Warren*: I haven't considered this. We have a
lot of things to do. As far as the first question is
concerned, we believe, although we don't have proof
that ethidium bromide is mimicking transformation.
Ethidium bromide is a mutagen because it will, in
yeast, create petites that lack certain cytochromes.
It might create a frame shift mutation, but it might be
temporary because in these cells if you remove the
ethidium bromide the changes are reversible. I neglected to say that growth rate is inhibited by ethidium
bromide about 20 or 30%. It may be that circular DNA
exists in the nucleus and we'd like to think that it is
being affected by the ethidium bromide.

G. *Milo*: What is the biological half life of
ethidium bromide in the culture medium? If it was very
short, say, compared to MNNG; would you detect it? The
compound may be already biologically transformed by the
cell, therefore, it already would have elicited the
type of alteration in glycoprotein synthesis you are
observing in your system. Again I submit this phenomenon may be due only to a transitory malignant state
expressed by the cell in those stressed conditions in

24

the culture.

L. DeLuca, NIH: I have two questions. One is, do you have any idea whether the neuraminidase levels of your transformed and normal cells are the same, or different? And, is the increase for peak B that you have mentioned in one case, a constant finding in your media from transformed cells and if so, if you are in fact releasing more of the B peak, would A to B ratio not increase, and therefore, your peak A look much bigger than it really is?

L. Warren: This puzzles us. I don't know what the explanation for that is but the A to B ratio looks constant in the cell no matter what you do, despite the fact that the protein you see in the medium, I think Susie talked about this, too...is primarily B glycopeptide. I have no explanation for it.

L. DeLuca: How about differences in neuraminidase level?

L. Warren: Well, we've looked and it's so feeble and variable I wouldn't want to make any generalizations. I don't think you can come to a conclusion about it.

B. Sanford, NIH: Is there any possibility that with the non-dividing cell the reason you're not seeing peak A material in the membrane is that this material is turning over rapidly and accumulating in the medium?

L. Warren: Well, we don't see it in the medium.

B. Sanford: You don't...

L. Warren: It may be destroyed. You see, when a cell turns over, the material can be destroyed within the cell, it can go out and be found in the medium, it can go out and come back...it's a very complicated thing. I don't know...it would take a lot of work to find out.

S. Roseman, Johns Hopkins University: I didn't get the comment about specificity. Do you think you have a specific sialyltransferase? What type is it with respect to the glycoproteins since there are at least two that we know of. Have you looked at that?

L. Warren: Well, I can say that it changes upon transformation whereas transferase activity to other acceptors do not change, second of all, transferase activity when we use desialated proteins of various kinds does not change. If we keep the enzyme preparation at 4 degrees in the refrigerator it seems that transferase activity of desialated peak A dies out but the transfer to the endogenous acceptor whose structure is actually unknown, we don't know what it's transferring to there, keeps going. There are no metal ion requirements...and it has a pH optimum of about 6.9...I neglected to say that we've done all the usual kinetics and have found linearity with time and with enzyme concentration, CNPNAN and acceptor concentration and so on.

S. Roseman: Does detergent affect the activity at all?

L. Warren: They inhibit considerably.

S. Roseman: The last question is, have you tried converting peak B to A by putting sialic acid on?

L. Warren: Well, that slide that I flashed by showed peak B as an acceptor. It accepts sialic acid but equally using control and transformed cell enzymes whereas, with the desialated A there was a three-fold difference in activity.

THE MECHANISM OF ENZYMATIC HALOGENATION AND ITS RELATION TO THE LABELING OF CELL SURFACE STRUCTURES*

Lowell P. Hager

Department of Biochemistry
University of Illinois
Urbana, Illinois   61801

The use of lactoperoxidase and radioisotopes of iodine has been widely adopted as a mechanism for cell surface and membrane labeling since its introduction by Morrison and co-workers. In our laboratory we have been engaged in studying the mechanism of enzymatic halogenation, mostly using chloroperoxidase as our model system. However, we feel certain that our findings with chloroperoxidase can be generalized to cover the broad spectrum of peroxidases which can catalyze halogenation reactions.

It becomes especially important to consider the mechanism of enzymatic halogenation when responding to the concerns of those who are using the lactoperoxidase catalyzed iodination reaction for detecting differences between normal and transformed cells. For example, in a previous session one of the speakers questioned whether or not elemental iodine (or I_3^-) was the actual iodinating species or whether an enzyme-bound electrophilic iodinating species was involved. Similarly, Dr. Phillip Robbins questioned whether or not there could be a specific interaction between lactoperoxidase and certain cell surface glycoproteins which could lead to extensive labeling of one or two types of surface glycoproteins while the reaction ignored other surface glycoproteins. A consideration of the mechanism of

* This research has been supported by grants from the National Institutes of Health (USPH RG 7768) and the National Science Foundation (NSF GB 30758X).

halogenation and of the specificities and kinds of peroxidases available for iodination reactions suggests direct experimentation to answer these questions.

The general halogenation reaction catalyzed by peroxidase is shown in equation 1.

$$X^- + H_2O_2 + Acceptor\text{-}H \rightarrow Acceptor\text{-}X + OH^- + H_2O \qquad (1)$$

In equation 1, X^- represents an oxidizable halogen anion (iodide, bromide or chloride). The peroxidases show broad specificity with respect to the halogen acceptor molecule. With chloroperoxidase, almost any good nucleophile will function as an acceptor. Tyrosine residues, either free or in peptide linkage are reasonably good acceptors and, of course, the tyrosine reaction is the important reaction in the glycoprotein labeling studies. The greatest complication is the fact that halogen anions themselves are good nucleophiles and therefore can compete with tyrosine residues as acceptors in the reaction (equation 2). In this case, the elemental halogen species is

$$2\ X^- + H_2O_2 \rightarrow X_2 + 2\ OH^- \qquad (2)$$

generated which can subsequently halogenate tyrosine residues; since the elemental halogen is a rapidly diffusing and membrane soluble species it could possibly penetrate membranes and label interior structures. This undoubtedly means that caution must be used and reaction conditions must be established in order to minimize the reaction leading to elemental halogen and maximize the tyrosine halogenation reaction.

Before turning to the discussion of mechanism, I want to briefly note the availability of different enzymes and radioactive halogen isotopes for labeling reactions. The question of labeling specific structures through peroxidase complexes could be studied by comparing surface iodination using different enzymes. Apparently all the heme peroxidases are capable of oxidizing iodide ion, thus, in addition to lactoperoxidase, horseradish peroxidase, chloroperoxidase, myleoperoxidase and yeast cytochrome c peroxidase are potential candidates for labeling surface components with iodine. Both horse-

28

radish and lactoperoxidase are commerically available and chloroperoxidase will soon be available on the commercial market. Chloroperoxidase and myleoperoxidase can also utilize bromide and chloride for enzymatic halogenation, thus extending the labeling reaction to ^{77}Br and ^{36}Cl. Bromine-77 is a short-lived gamma emitter and is useful for protein labeling in clinical studies (1); however, it does not appear to be of particular use in studies on cell surface labeling. On the other hand, ^{36}Cl could be quite useful as a surface structure label. Chlorine-36 is a β-emitter, about 7 times more powerful than ^{14}C, and has a long half-life. Other than the fact that the long half-life means relatively low specific activity, ^{36}Cl lends itself to labeling when isolation of the labeled compound(s) is undertaken. The stability of the radioactive label in this case is an important considera-tion.

During the past several years studies in our labora-tory on chloroperoxidase and the mechanism of enzymatic halogenation suggest that halogenation proceeds through and enzyme-bound halogenating intermediate which is formed by the reaction of peroxidase Compound I with halide anions (2-4). The reaction sequence can be formulated as shown in equation 3-6.

$$\text{Native enzyme} + H_2O_2 \rightarrow \text{Compound I} \qquad (3)$$
$$\text{Compound I} + X^- \rightarrow \text{Enzyme} - X^+ \qquad (4)$$
$$\text{Enzyme-}X^+ + \text{Acceptor} \rightarrow \text{Enzyme-}X^+\text{-Acceptor} \qquad (5)$$
$$\text{Enzyme-}X^+ - \text{Acceptor} \rightarrow \text{Acceptor-}X + \text{Native enzyme} \qquad (6)$$

Compound I appears to be a common intermediate in all peroxidase reactions and is derived from the interaction of the native enzyme with hydrogen peroxide. Early studies (5) showed that Compound I contains the two oxidizing equivalents associated with hydrogen peroxide and recent studies in our laboratory have shown that one and only one atom of oxygen from hydrogen peroxide is incorporated into Compound I (6-8). The findings to-gether with the studies of Dolphin, Felton and co-workers (9) on the structure of oxidize cobalt-porphyrin com-pounds suggest a hydroxyl ligand on a Fe^{+4} -porphyrin cation radical species (Fig. 1) as the most appropriate structure for Compound I. We have suggested that the

formation of the halogenating intermediate from Compound
I involves the replacement of hydroxyl ligand with a
hypohalite ligand (OCl, OBr or OI) and that this intermediate is the active halogenating species (Fig. 1). In
this formulation, the iron atom in the iron protoporphyrin
IX returns to the Fe^{+3} in the halogenating intermediate
and the oxidizing equivalents of Compound I are formally
associated with the hypohalite ligand.

In support of this suggestion we have recently found
that both chloroperoxidase and horseradish peroxidase will
react with chlorite ($NaClO_2$) and form a chlorinating
intermediate without going through a Compound I intermediate (10). In addition to being an important contribution to the mechanism problem, the chlorite reaction
offers an alternative substrate for cell surface labeling
studies. Radioactively labeled chlorite ($Na^{36}ClO_2$) can
be readily prepared and since a free halide anion is
not required in the reaction, there is no opportunity
for the enzyme to generate elemental chlorine and thus
complicate the labeling reaction. In addition, since
both horseradish and chloroperoxidase are capable of
utilizing chlorite, it is probably safe to predict that
other peroxidases will also utilize this substrate for
enzymatic chlorination. The chloroperoxidase and
horseradish peroxidase reactions with chlorite extend
over a broad pH profile (pH 2.5 to 7) and thus offer a
wide range of reaction conditions for labeling studies.

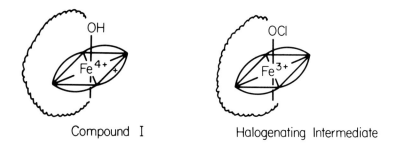

Compound I   Halogenating Intermediate

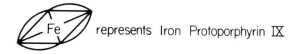 represents Iron Protoporphyrin IX

Fig. 1.   Suggested Structures for Compound I and the Halogenating Intermediate.

REFERENCES

1. Knight, L., Krohn, K.A., Welch, M.J., Spomer, W.E., and Hager, L.P., Bromine-77: A New Protein Label, Proc. of International Conference on Radiopharmaceuticals, Soc. of Nuclear Medicine, February, 1974.

2. Morris, D.R., and Hager, L.P., J. Biol. Chem. 241, 1763 (1966).

3. Hager, L.P., Morris, D.R., Brown, F.S., and Eberwein, H., J. Biol. Chem. 241, 1769 (1966).

4. Brown, F.S., and Hager, L.P., J. Am. Chem. Soc. 89, 719 (1967).

5. Chance, B., Arch. Biochem. Biophys. 22, 224 (1949).

6. Hager, L.P., Doubek, D.L., Silverstein, R.M., Hargis, J.H. and Martin, J.C., J. Am. Chem. Soc. 94, 4364 (1972).

7. Hager, L.P., Doubek, D.L., Silverstein, R.M., Lee, T.T., Thomas, J.A., Hargis, J.H. and Martin, J.C. in "Oxidases and Related Redox Systems", T.E. King, H.S. Mason and M. Morrison, Editors, p. 311 (1973).

8. Hager, L.P., Doubek, D.L. and Hollenberg, P. in "The Molecular Basis of Electron Transport (Miami Winter Symposium, Vol. 4), p. 347 (1972).

9. Dolphin, D., Forman, A., Borg, D.C., Fajer, J. and Felton, R.H., Proc. Nat. Acad. Sci. 68, 614 (1971).

10. Hollenberg, P., Meir, T. and Hager, L.P. Submitted to the J. Biol. Chem. (1974).

THE USE OF LACTOPEROXIDASE AS A
MOLECULAR AND MACROMOLECULAR PROBE

MARTIN MORRISON, RONALD E. GATES and C. THOMAS HUBER
Laboratory of Biochemistry
St. Jude Children's Research Hospital
Memphis, Tennessee 38101

Abstract: The properties of lactoperoxidase which make
the iodination reaction catalyzed by this enzyme suitable for use as a molecular and macromolecular probe
are discussed. Some of the limitations and precautions in the applications of these probes are pointed
out. Examples are given of the use of lactoperoxidase
labeling as membrane marker in isolation procedures.

A study of the exposed proteins of human lymphoblasts
and lymphocytes is given which demonstrates the use
of double labeling method on small quantities of whole
cells.

The enzyme, lactoperoxidase, can be used as both a
molecular and macromolecular probe. These uses are based
upon its properties as an enzyme. Our studies (1,2) of
the mechanisms of lactoperoxidase catalyzed iodination
indicate that lactoperoxidase rapidly catalyzes the oxidation of iodide, as do all hemoprotein peroxidases.
Iodine (I_2) produced by such a reaction at neutral pH
values will react with phenolic compounds to give iodinated
derivatives. Thus, by this mechanism all peroxidases can
be considered to catalyze iodination. In fact, they
simply catalyze the oxidation of iodide. In contrast to
this mechanism, lactoperoxidase does not catalyze the
iodination of tyrosine via I_2. This is a most important

33

point in the use of this enzyme as a probe.

The mechanism of catalysis probably follows the classical George Chance scheme for peroxidases, and one mole of peroxide is consumed per mole of iodide incorporated into tyrosine. Lactoperoxidase forms an enzyme substrate complex with the iodinatable substrates in this enzyme catalyzed reaction. The enzyme itself probably catalyzes the ionization of the phenolic group to form a phenolate ion which is the species attacked in the enzyme catalyzed iodination.

An enzyme with these properties can be used as a tool, a molecular probe, to analyze the structure of proteins. Since the enzyme catalyzes iodination of only those tyrosine residues with which it can complex, the enzyme will iodinate selectively only those residues available by virtue of their geometric position. Those groups will be iodinated which can complex with the enzyme. Thus, iodination via the enzyme will establish the geometric location of tyrosine residues within a molecule. Other methods of iodinating proteins are also selective but give results based on the chemical reactivity of the tyrosine residue and not its geometric location. Any group which is iodinated by lactoperoxidase must have been accessible to the enzyme. Our studies of cytochrome c illustrate this point (1,3). Horse heart cytochrome c contains 4 tyrosine residues. Chemical iodination procedures have established that two of these residues, residue 67 and 74, are iodinated (4,5). X-ray data (6) showed that residue 67 is buried in the hydrophobic core of the molecule even though it is the most readily iodinated of the two residues. With enzymatic iodination only residue 74 is iodinated (3).

The enzymatic method of iodination is very sensitive and allows us to test conformational changes in the protein. Oxidized cytochrome c is readily iodinated and as many as two moles of iodide can be incorporated per mole of cytochrome c. Reduction of the cytochrome c gives a conformational change which alters the accessibility of the tyrosine residue 74, and in this state the protein is not iodinated with lactoperoxidase (6).

Recently, Dickerson et al. (6,7) showed that in reduced cytochrome c the aromatic ring of tyrosine residue
74 moves with respect to the backbone of the molecule.
This relatively small change in position of the side
chain of the tyrosine residue alters its accessibility
to the lactoperoxidase and it is not iodinated. From
this it is clear that lactoperoxidase can be used to
study the position of a particular tyrosine residue in a
protein. Further, this method can be used as a probe
for conformational changes which result in altered
accessibility of tyrosine residues to lactoperoxidase.

Lactoperoxidase can also be used as a unique probe for
the vectorial arrangement of membrane proteins, that is,
as a macromolecular probe (1,8,9). The enzyme has a high
molecular weight of 78,600 and does not dissociate into
subunits (9). Hence, it does not readily penetrate an
intact membrane. Almost all proteins which have been
studied can be iodinated, and although they are iodinated
at different rates, the differences in these rates are
less than one order of magnitude (2,10). Membrane proteins labeled with this system must be present on the
surface exposed to the lactoperoxidase, since only
those proteins to which the enzyme has access will be
iodinated. The vectorial arrangement of proteins in any
membrane can therefore be determined with this probe.

Our studies with normal human erythrocytes illustrate
this use of the enzyme. Although the membrane contains
about 20 polypeptides, only a 90,000 dalton protein,
as well as the major and two minor glycoproteins are
labeled on the external surface (8,9,11). On the other
hand, when the enzyme is accessible to both sides of the
membrane, almost all the membrane proteins are iodinated.
Thus, most of the membrane protein was found to be on the
interior surface.

Since our initial work many investigators have applied
this method to studies of a variety of membrane structures
and cell types (12-20). The procedure has some practi-
cal limitations which have not always been recognized (21). It is necessary to be certain the membrane
under study is intact. Broken membranes will allow the
enzyme access to both sides of the membrane. Further,

soluble proteins are iodinated more readily than membrane bound proteins. When the membrane is broken no definitive information on vectorial position of proteins can be obtained.

As pointed out above, peroxidases can generate iodine, I_2. Iodine can readily pass through membranes and will react with lipids by adding across double bands. It will also react with phenolic groups of proteins in a non-enzyme catalyzed reaction. Thus, iodination resulting from iodine (I_2) gives no information concerning the arrangement of membrane proteins. In order to avoid the production of iodine (I_2), low concentrations of iodide should be employed, and excess iodinatable substrate should be present.

While this approach has been widely used to identify exposed membrane proteins, it also provides a valuable way of characterizing membrane preparations. Any isolated membrane reflects the techniques employed to isolate it. For most membranes serious problems are involved in removing extraneous proteins and other subcellular organelles and membranes. The purity of a membrane system is usually determined by the use of enzyme markers. Unfortunately, the use of enzymes to characterize a membrane may give rise to ambiguous results (see 22,23 for recent reviews). The enzyme marker must be tightly associated with only the membrane in question, but the arguments used to establish this are often circular. Furthermore, the activity of an enzyme does not depend only on the amount of enzyme. It also depends on the presence of inhibitors or activators which may be added or lost during membrane isolation. Indeed, enzyme activity can be changed by denaturing or disorganizing the membrane during isolation.

Radioactive iodide incorporated into a membrane by lactoperoxidase catalyzed iodination is an ideal membrane marker. The radioactivity is covalently linked to only those proteins accessible to lactoperoxidase, i.e., exposed membrane proteins of a cell or isolated organelle. Therefore, this marker is unambiguously associated with the membrane. Furthermore, the assay for the marker is both convenient and very sensitive, since

gamma emissions from the iodine isotope are readily
detected and quantitated. The iodine label then provides
a means of following the fate of the membrane in any
fractionation procedure. The amount of label per mg
protein gives an index of the extent of purification. This
method has been used in our laboratory to follow the purification of plasma membrane preparations from Ehrlich
ascites tumor cells (1,24) and platelets (25),and the
outer membrane of mitochondria (26).

While purity is the simplest parameter for characterizing a membrane preparation, an equally important
question is whether the total membrane has been isolated
or only certain fragments of the membrane. Loss of membrane proteins can be ascertained by determining the
ratio of various labeled components in the whole preparation with the ratio obtained in the isolated fractions.
If the ratios are not identical for all the labeled
components, then selective loss of membrane proteins has
occurred. This same approach can be used with enzyme
markers, but several enzyme markers may not be known for
a given membrane. With the lactoperoxidase probe system
generally a number of proteins are always labeled,
therefore providing multiple membrane markers. The
isolation of membranes was followed with this procedure
in Ehrlich ascitestumor cells (24) and platelets (25).
The isolated membrane had the same components in the same
ratio as whole cells. Therefore, there was no evidence
for loss of proteins during membrane isolation.

With the outer membrane from mitochondria a different
result was obtained. Intact mitochondria from rat liver
were labeled by the lactoperoxidase iodination method
(26). The integrity of the outer membrane was established before and after iodination of the intact
mitochondria by assay of adenylate kinase, a soluble
intermembrane enzyme.

After isolation of the outer membrane from labeled
intact mitochondria by a mild digitonin procedure and
purification of the membrane by differential centrifugation, the specific radioactivity of the iodine marker
increased twelve-fold. It is interesting that the
labeling pattern obtained after separation of polypeptides

of the outer membrane fraction by SDS gel electrophoresis indicated that 70% of the total iodine label was in components of the 14,000 molecular weight region. The pattern observed for the intact mitochondria had a lower percentage of these labeled components. In addition, the fragments of outer membrane remaining with the inner membrane-matrix fraction showed several higher molecular weight species with a much larger degree of labeling relative to the 14,000 region than was observed with the outer membrane fraction.

Since the outer membrane fragments isolated showed a different distribution of iodine label among the various molecular weight classes than did outer membrane fragments remaining with the inner membrane-matrix particles, it was suggested that these correspond to separate regions of a heterogeneous membrane.

This finding may be significant in regard to Hackenbrock's (27) observation of contact points between the outer and inner mitochondrial membrane. It is possible that the region of the outer membrane at the contact points remained with the inner membrane-matrix fraction after digitonin fractionation. This concept is depicted in Fig. 1 which shows the outer membrane fracture occurring in a manner such that fragments rich in higher molecular weight iodinatable components (shown as black geometric shapes) remain with the inner membrane-matrix particle. These outer membrane fragments may adhere to the inner membrane-matrix particle because they are located at the points of contact between the outer and inner membrane. Those outer membrane fragments which are dislodged from the mitochondrion by the digitonin treatment are rich in the 14,000 iodinatable polypeptides shown as white geometric shapes.

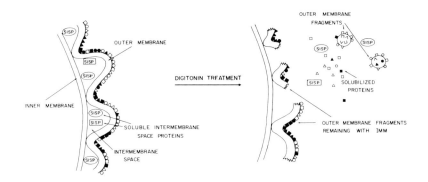

Fig. 1. Scheme for the fragmentation of the outer mitochondrial membrane by digitonin treatment. A scheme depicting the distribution of mitochondrial membrane components following digitonin treatment of rat liver mitochondria. The iodinatable components of the outer membrane are shown as various geometric shapes, both black and white, attached to the outer membrane. As a result of the digitonin treatment the outer membrane is broken releasing soluble inter-membrane space proteins (SISP), outer membrane frag-ments, soluble proteins and inner membrane-matrix particles. Portions of the outer membrane remain with the inner membrane.

Finally, since the subject of this symposia is membrane glycoprotein and cancer, we would like to present some data pertinent to this topic obtained with the lactoperoxidase probe system. Proteins exposed on the surface of human lymphoblasts (CCRF-CEM) and lymphocytes were iodinated using lactoperoxidase. The lymphoblasts were derived from a patient with acute lymphocytic leukemia and main-tained in cell culture while the lymphocytes were isolated from normal human peripheral blood. Each of these cell types was labeled with the lactoperoxidase system. Since

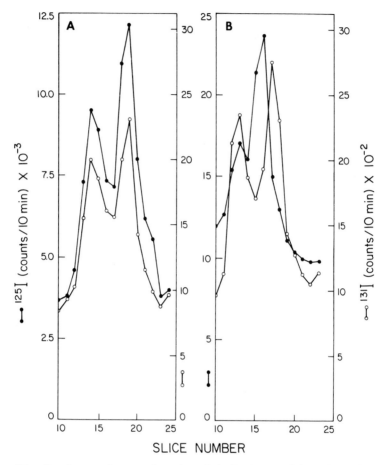

Fig.2. Comparison of major labeled peptides from leukemic lymphoblasts and normal lymphocytes. The distribution of the major radioactive labeled peptides on SDS-acrylamide gels is shown. 2A demonstrates the sensitivity of the double labeling technique. It shows that identical patterns are obtained when lymphoblasts are labeled with ^{125}I or ^{131}I and analyzed on the same gel. 2B demonstrates the difference in exposed peptides on the surface of leukemic lymphoblasts and normal lymphocytes. It shows the patterns when ^{131}I labeled lymphoblasts and ^{125}I labeled lymphocytes are analyzed in this way on the same gel.

small quantities of material were available we could not
actually study the isolated plasma membrane, but we did
devise a method for handling the whole cells. After
labeling, the cells were heated to 100° C for 3 min.,
incubated with DNAase, solubilized in SDS and peptides
separated on SDS-acrylamide gels.

In order to compare the closely related cell types we
have employed a double labeling technique. The two
different cell samples were labeled with different isotopes of iodine, ^{125}I or ^{131}I. Following solubilization,
the samples were mixed and proteins were separated by
electrophoresis on the same gel. The gel was sliced and
the amount of each isotope in the slices determined with
a double channel gamma spectrometer. This approach is
extremely powerful for resolving small differences between
labeled peptides because all differences due to sample
preparation, gel electrophoresis or gel slicing are
eliminated. Figure 2A is a control which shows how well
the double labeling technique works. One half of a
lymphoblast preparation was labeled with ^{125}I while the
other half was labeled with ^{131}I. Following solubilization the samples were mixed and electrophoresed on the
same gel. It is obvious that the labeling patterns are
identical for the region of the gel shown in Figure 2A.
This region shows the two major labeled peptides present
on the entire gel. The smaller peak has a molecular
weight of 120,000 daltons, while the larger is 105,000
daltons. When lymphocytes were labeled with ^{125}I and
lymphoblasts with ^{131}I, and the proteins separated by
electrophoresis, the results shown in Figure 2B were
obtained. The labeling patterns are not identical. The
smaller peak in each case has a molecular weight of
120,000 daltons, while the larger peak is 110,000 daltons
in lymphocytes and 105,000 daltons in lymphoblasts. We
conclude that at least one major exposed protein on the
surface of these two cell types is different. Preliminary
data indicate that the 105,000 dalton labeled peptide in
lymphoblasts is altered on neuraminidase treatment of intact cells. Therefore, this component may be a glycoprotein. The difference between normal lymphocytes and
leukemic lymphoblasts seen in Figure 2B may be due to
different amounts of sialic acid on the glycoprotein. Such
differences in sialic acid content between normal and tumor
cells have been reported (28, 29,30). The relationship

41

of the difference between normal lymphocytes and leukemic lymphoblasts seen in Figure 2B to sialic levels and the oncogenic process is being investigated.

This work was supported in part by USPHS Grants GM 15913 and CA 13534.

REFERENCES

(1) M. Morrison and R.E. Gates, in: The Molecular Basis of Electron Transport, ed. by J. Schultz and B. E. Cameron, Academic Press, New York (1972) p. 327.

(2) M. Morrison and G. Bayse in: Oxidases and Related Redox Systems, ed. by Tsoo E. King, Howard S. Mason and Martin Morrison, University Park Press, Baltimore (1973) p. 375.

(3) E. Margoliash, S. Ferguson-Miller, J. Tulloss, C.H. Kang, B.A. Feinberg, D.L. Brautigan and M. Morrison, Proc. Nat. Acad. Sci. 70 (1973) 3245.

(4) E. B. McGowan and E. Stellwagen, Biochemistry 9 (1970) 3047.

(5) K. Naritz, K. Sugeno, T. Mizoguchi and K. Hamaguchi in: Structure and Function of Cytochromes, ed. by K. Okunuki, M.D. Kamen and I. Sukuzu, University Park Press, Baltimore (1968) p. 1362.

(6) R. E. Dickerson, T. Takano, D. Eisenberg, O. B. Kallai, L. Samson, A. Cooper and E. Margoliash, J. Biol. Chem. 246 (1971) 1511.

(7) T. Takano, O. B. Kallai, R. Swanson and R. E. Dickerson, J. Biol. Chem. 248 (1973) 5234.

(8) D. R. Phillips, and M. Morrison, Biochem. Biophys. Res. Commun. 40 (1970) 284.

(9) D. R. Phillips and M. Morrison, Biochemistry 10 (1971) 1766.

(10) M.Morrison, Gunma Symposia on Endocrinology 5 (1968) 239.

(11) M.Morrison, T. Mueller and C. T. Huber, J. Biol. Chem. (In Press).

(12) J.F. Poduslo, C.S. Greenberg and M.C. Glick, Biochemistry 11 (1972) 2616.

(13) J.W. Uhr, and E.S. Vitetta, Fed. Proc. 32 (1973) 35.

(14) J. J. Marchalonis, R. E. Cone and V. Santer, Biochem. J. 124 (1971) 921.

(15) S. J. Kennel and R. A. Lerner, J. Mol. Biol. 76 (1973) 485.

(16) M.P. Czech, and W.S. Lynn, Biochemistry 12 (1973) 3597.

(17) R.O. Hynes, Proc. Nat. Acad. Sci. 70 (1973) 3170.

(18) B. C. Shin, and K. L. Carraway, Biochim. Biophys. Acta 330 (1973) 254.

(19) G. Kreibich, and D. D. Sabatini, Fed. Proc. 32 (1973) 2133.

(20) C. J. Michalski, B.H. Sells, and M. Morrison, Eur. J. Biochem. 33 (1973) 481.

(21) M. Morrison, Methods in Enzymology, Vol. 32 B Academic Press, New York (In Press).

(22) J.W. DePierre and M. L. Karnovsky, J. Cell Biol. 56 (1973) 275.

(23) D.F.H. Wallach and P.S. Lin, Biochim. Biophys.Acta 300 (1973) 211.

(24) R.E. Gates, M. McClain and M. Morrison, Exper. Cell Res. (In Press).

(25) D. R. Phillips, Biochemistry 11 (1972) 4582.

(26) C.T. Huber and M. Morrison, Biochemistry 12 (1973) 4274.

(27) C. R. Hackenbrock, Proc. Nat. Acad. Sci. 61 (1968) 598.

(28) W. P. Van Beek, L. A. Smets, and P. Emmelot, Cancer Res. 33 (1973) 2913.

(29) L. Warren, J. P. Fuhrer, and C.A. Buck, Proc. Nat. Acad. Sci. 69 (1972) 1838.

(30) M. C. Glick, Z. Rabinowitz and L. Sachs, Biochemistry 12 (1973) 4864.

DISCUSSION

W. Lands, University of Michigan: I'd like to ask Dr. Morrison about the experiment in which he got no labeling of the reduced cytochrome c. I want to know if you are implying that the tyrosine is not available to the iodinating enzyme. A second interpretation would be that the conditions used to prepare and maintain the reduced cytochrome c in the reaction mixture were suffici- ent to prevent your lactoperoxidase from functioning at all. It would be quite important to show that there was indeed iodination of another protein in that same reaction mixture in which cytochrome c is not being iodinated. Do you have that kind of control? I just want to know whether the controls show that your enzyme is still capable of functioning.

M. Morrison, St. Jude Children's Research Hospital: Oh, yes, our enzymes are perfectly capable of functioning. Cytochrome c is non-auto-oxidizable so you can reduce it and prepare it free of reducing agents. It's perfectly capable of staying that way for a reasonable period of time.

W. Lands: Is my question reasonably clear to you? Have you actually done an experiment where you did iodinate a protein in the presence of reduced cytochrome c?

M. Morrison: I haven't done that exact experiment. I can assure you that there's nothing in the cytochrome c that would inhibit iodination of another protein.

M. Sherman: I'd like to ask Dr. Hager a question. Does the use of chlorite (ClO^-_2) shift the pH optimum of the chloroperoxidase reaction to a value more suitable for work with cells?

45

L. P. Hager, University of Illinois: Not for chloroperoxidase, but horseradish peroxidase utilizes chlorite quite effectively. The pH optimum for horseradish peroxidase is about pH 4.5, however, horseradish peroxidase is quite effective in the pH range of 6 as well. I would suspect as I said in the talk, we haven't tested lactoperoxidase, but I would expect a more favorable pH for the chlorite reaction also with lactoperoxidase.

M. Sherman: Thank you.

I. Fritz, University of Toronto: I was very interested in the mitochondrial experiments. What portions of the inner membrane particles were iodinated by the lactoperoxidase system when intact mitochondria were employed? Did you identify which specific protein or enzyme was labeled in the other part of the experiment. When you stripped off the outer membrane first, did you get the same type of protein in the isolated inner membrane particle that you observed when intact mitochondria were incubated with lactoperoxidase?

M. Morrison: We haven't completely identified all of the iodinated proteins. We're in the process of doing that. If you strip off and then iodinate the outer membrane, then the same molecular weight classes of proteins are iodinated as well as the other proteins made accessible by opening the membrane.

I. Fritz: Can you rule out the possibility that you had iodinated outer membrane proteins which then reattached to the inner membrane particle during the procedure of stripping off the outer membranes?

M. Morrison: No, what we are saying is that with this method we label the outer membrane components, but when we strip away the outer membrane we do not remove all the labeled components. Some specific proteins stick with the inner membrane. These proteins may be at contact points between the inner and outer membrane. Without this labeling method these proteins might be considered part of the inner membrane, since they remain with the inner membrane in the fractionation procedure.

V. P. Hollander, Hospital for Joint Diseases: Dr. Morrison, how much radioactivity would be introduced in your system by virtue of iodination of the lactoperoxidase itself which then might be hard to separate from some other product?

M. Morrison: Lactoperoxidase can be iodinated. You can put in more than 3 moles of iodine per mole of lacto-peroxidase before it loses appreciable amounts of its activity. Specifically, to answer your question, it would depend upon how much lactoperoxidase was added. In most cases such small amounts of the enzyme are added compared to other proteins that it should not be very significant. Most commercial preparations of the enzyme are far from pure and have many contaminating proteins. These proteins would also, of course, be iodinated and may present some difficulties.

J. Wolff, National Institutes of Health: Is there evidence that the interaction of the enzyme with the acceptor is merely of an entropic nature, that is just binding, or is there some kind of activation of the substrate as well? Second question, what happens to the histidines in your cytochrome c system?

L. P. Hager: I can respond to the first question, the evidence for reaction step three, that is a formation of a complex between the halogenating intermediate and an acceptor is based on kinetic studies. If you try and do binding studies by measuring the binding of an acceptor to the enzyme, through equilibrium dialysis, you always get negative results. However in the equilibrium dialysis studies when you do binding by equilibrium dialysis you're looking at the native enzyme and not the halogenating intermediate. I think we have to rely on the evidence from kinetic studies which would say that there is a specific binding between acceptor and the halogenating intermediate once its formed.

J. Wolff: But is it only binding or is it electron abstraction or something in addition?

L. P. Hager: No, I believe its only binding.

M. Morrison: You will recall the work of Dunford in "Oxidases and Related Redox Systems," ed. by Kind, T. F., Mason, H. S. and Morrison, M., Univ. Park Press, Baltimore, (1973) p. 366, which suggests that there is binding of cresol, which can be thought of as a tyrosine derivative, to horseradish peroxidase (HRP) and the binding constant indicated that one mole of cresol was bound to each mole of enzyme. The data also indicated that cresol binds ten times more tightly to Compound II than to native HRP. Oxidation of cresol takes place in this case giving coupling. We have studied that coupling with tyrosine and in both HRP and lactoperoxidase there is stereo specific coupling (BBA 284: 34 (1972), Oxidases and Related Redox Systems, ed. by King, Mason and Morrison, University Park Press, Baltimore (1973) p. 375).

L. P. Hager: Yes, but the oxidation of the tyrosine is the first step, not the third step.

M. Morrison: Oh, yes, but I think that's what you were referring to, were you not?

L. P. Hager: Yes, for tyrosine oxidation, not for halogenation.

S. Roseman, Johns Hopkins University: It's really more in the nature of a comment. While everybody seems to be using this technique, the membrane proteins that we study have an extremely low content of tyrosine. In fact, we've gone away from using the Lowry method for determining protein in these cases. In fact, you may recall from Jeanloz's paper, that he reported an extremely low content of aromatic amino acids in that huge molecule that covers the surface of his cells; I don't think it had more than one tyrosine residue. So what I'm doing is questioning the reliability of the entire method for these proteins since it is based on tyrosine.

M. Morrison: Histidine would be iodinated. The method has limitations as do all methods, but that does not mean it is an unreliable procedure. The fact that certain proteins don't iodinate is a limitation, and I was trying to point those limitations out.

J. Schultz, Papanicolaou Cancer Research Institute:
The experiment you described with this charger where you
increase the peroxide concentration is confusing. You
know that when you add peroxide to a peroxidase system
that you get a bell-shaped curve when you plot the peroxide
concentration versus the velocity. And at the appex of
the curve it is practically stoichiometrical with the
amount of peroxide and enzyme, so if you increase the
peroxide concentration at one point, you should exceed
that appex and start getting inhibition where the peroxide
becomes a donor.

M. Morrison: I think we all agree that compound 4
could be produced at high concentrations of peroxidase and
this is an inactive form of the enzyme.

THE EXTERNAL PROTEINS OF HAMSTER CELLS AND THEIR VIRUS TRANSFORMED DERIVATIVES

RICHARD HYNES and IAN MACPHERSON
Department of Tumour Virology
Imperial Cancer Research Fund Laboratories
Lincoln's Inn Fields, London

Abstract: Proteins exposed at the surface of the NIL8 line of hamster cells have been identified by lactoperoxidase catalysed iodination (1). Several of these proteins comigrate with fucose and glucosamine labelled proteins. The main external protein, which appears to be glycosylated, is much reduced or missing in virus-transformed derivatives of NIL8 cells. It is very sensitive to tryptic digestion and is expressed maximally in dense cultures. The possibility that this protein has a role in the regulation of cell growth is discussed.

INTRODUCTION

The current concentration of studies on changes at the surface of transformed animal cells has shown the plasma membrane to be a complex organelle capable of accommodating a remarkable array of alterations. At present much of our information about these changes is descriptive and hypotheses on the regulation of cell growth based on key events at the cell surface are hard pressed to encompass the wide range of changes described.

Our studies have been concerned with the role of glycoproteins and glycosphingolipids at the cell surface in growth regulation. These molecules are potential receptor sites for signals from the medium and neighbouring cells.

Normal cells respond to high population density and the depletion of serum growth factors by entering a quiescent or "holding" condition in the post mitotic or early G1 phase of the cell cycle. A consistent property of transformed cells is their immunity from these restraints.

Certain stable cell lines retain a normal response to these restraints and the study described here makes use of such a line of Syrian hamster cells viz. NIL8, a variant clone derived from the NIL2 line (2). It has a low saturation density even in the presence of serum concentrations in excess of 5%.

Derivatives transformed by infection with polyoma virus or hamster sarcoma virus (HSV) (3) have been isolated from colonies growing in agar suspension culture.

The relevance of this work to cancer biology is that the normal cell block in the G1 phase is presumably an in vitro expression of an in vivo homeostatic control which a potential cancer cell must overcome in order to give rise to a neoplastic focus.

IODINATION OF SURFACE PROTEINS OF NIL8 CELLS

The technique of lactoperoxidase - catalysed iodination attaches ^{125}I covalently to proteins via their tyrosine residues. When applied to cells in culture the large molecular weight of the lactoperoxidase and glucose oxidase molecules used in the reaction (see legend to Fig. 1) should theoretically prevent their passage through the plasma membrane thus ensuring that only proteins at the cell surface are labelled.

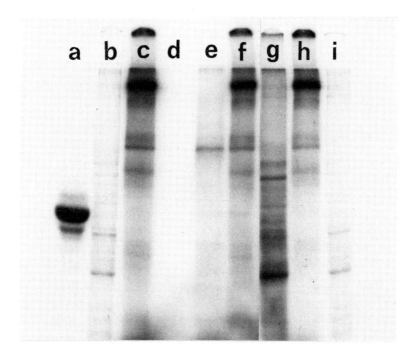

Fig. 1. Iodination of NIL8 cells. Autoradiogram of 7.5% SDS-polyacrylamide slab gel. (a) iodinated calf serum; (b and i) cells labelled with ^{14}C-leucine-3 days; (c and h) cells iodinated in monolayer; (d) cells iodinated as in c minus enzymes (e) cells iodinated and then treated for 10 min with 10µg/ml trypsin (f) cells iodinated then treated with 10µg/ml trypsin + 10µg/ml of soyabean trypsin inhibitor; (g) cells lysed with water then iodinated. All iodinated samples contained equal quantities of protein.

Cultures in Petri dishes were washed three times with phosphate buffered saline pH-7.2 and labelled in buffer containing 5mM glucose, 400μCi/ml carrier-free sodium ^{125}I-iodide, 20μg/ml lactoperoxidase and 0.1 U/ml glucose oxidase for 10 min at room temperature. The reaction was stopped by adding phosphate buffered sodium iodide (PBI). The cells were scraped into PBI containing 2mM phenyl methyl sulphonyl fluoride (PMSF a protease inhibitor), centrifuged and dissolved by boiling in electrophoresis sample buffer containing 2% SDS and 2mM PMSF. Samples were made 0.1 M with dithiothreitol and boiled again before electrophoresis.

Figure 1 shows autoradiograph of a 7.5% SDS-polyacrylamide slab gel in which the proteins of NIL8 cells labelled by iodination (Fig. 1 c and h) are compared with similar cultures labelled for 3 days with ^{14}C-leucine (Fig. 1 b and i). It is clear that many of the proteins present in the metabolically labelled (^{14}C-leucine) tracks are absent from the iodinated preparation. This is also apparent in disc gel preparations of similarly labelled preparations. Omission of either enzyme or glucose from the reaction prevents iodination (Fig. 1 d). In preparations from NIL8 cells lysed with water and then iodinated the labelling pattern resembles that of cells metabolically labelled with ^{14}C-leucine indicating that the proteins which were not labelled in the iodinated living cells were unavailable. (cf. Figs. 1 g, h and i).

The pattern of iodinated calf serum proteins (Fig. 1a) is distinct from that of the whole cells (Fig. 1 c and h) showing that the surface proteins accepting the iodine label are not derived from serum proteins bound to the cells. Also cells grown in iodinated calf serum did not bind labelled proteins to their surface. At least two lines of evidence support the belief that the selectivity of the iodine labelling of the NIL8 cells is the result of the reaction affecting only proteins at the cell surface. Firstly, a brief treatment of the iodinated cells with a dilute solution (10μg/ml) of trypsin at room temperature results in the loss of all but one of the iodinated proteins indicating that they are available at the cell surface (Fig. 1 e). Soyabean trypsin inhibitor blocks the action of the trypsin (Fig. 1 f) showing that it is acting as a protease. Secondly when iodinated NIL8 cells were homogenised by nitrogen cavitation and the membrane vesicles separated by rate zonal centrifugation in dextran and sucrose gradients (4) the iodine label was predominantly in the membrane fraction. The highest specific activity was in fractions containing the plasma membrane enzyme markers, i.e. Na^+/K^+ stimulated Mg^{2+} ATPase and 5' nucleotidase activity. The nuclei and soluble proteins were not labelled. Thus it seems clear that the iodination procedure labels only proteins accessible at the cell surface and that these are cell derived.

THE CLONAL VARIATION OF IODINATED SURFACE PROTEINS IN NIL8 CELLS

Eight subclones of NIL8 had essentially similar patterns of iodinated proteins. Another clone derived from the parental stock of NIL2E cells, designated NIL clone 1 which has a more fibroblastic morphology and a higher saturation density than the NIL8 cells had an iodination pattern similar to that of NIL8.

Other cell lines studied included BHK21/13, 3T3, 3T6 and chicken embryo fibroblasts; these also have a major band and a number of lesser bands like NIL8 although they were individually distinct in detail and the distribution of the polypeptide bands.

CHARACTERISATION OF IODINATED NIL8 CELL PROTEINS

NIL8 cells incubated for 3 days with either ^{14}C-fucose (3μC/ml) or ^{14}C-glucosamine (5μC/ml) contained labelled glycoproteins which co-migrated in SDS-polyacrylamide gel electrophoresis with the major band(band 1) in iodinated preparations (5) (Fig. 2). Like the iodinated band the fucose and glucosamine labelled proteins were lost by mild trypsinisation (Fig. 2 b, d, h) and transformation (Fig. 2 c and i), which suggests that the protein detected as band 1 by iodination is identical with the glycoprotein of the same mobility which is labelled metabolically by sugars.

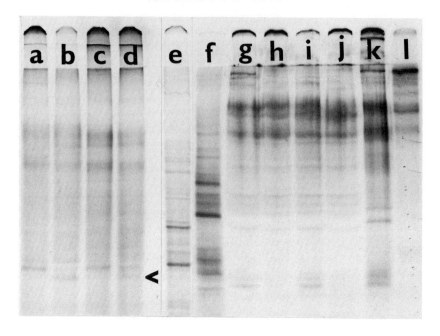

Fig. 2. Labelling of cells with ^{14}C-glucosamine and ^{14}C-fucose. Composite figure : autoradiographs of two gels (a-e) 7%, (f-1) 8%. Samples were labelled as follows (a-d) ^{14}C gluco-samine -5µC/ml for 3 days; (e-f) ^{14}C-leucine 1µC/ml 3 days; (g-j) ^{14}C-fucose 3µC/ml- 3 days, (k), ^{14}C-glucosamine 5µC/ml - 3 days. (l) iodinated. (c, d, i and j) - NIL8-HSV6, others NIL8. (b, d, h, and j) were treated with 10µg/ml trypsin for 10 min before harvesting for electrophoresis. The arrow marks the position of a glucosamine labelled band which appears after trypsin treatment of both "normal" and transformed cells.

No indication was obtained that the iodinated bands contained sulphated mucopolysaccharides or that they contain hyaluronic acid since they were not degraded by chondroitinase ABC or hyaluronidase nor were co-migrating bands obtained from cells labelled for 2 days with ^{35}S-sulphate (100µC/ml). Also preliminary evidence from proline labelling and co-migration experiments with α and β collagen preparations from calf skin and rat tail suggest that the iodinated proteins are not identical with collagen.

56

IODINATION OF SURFACE PROTEINS OF POLYOMA AND HAM-
STER SARCOMA VIRUS TRANSFORMED NIL8 CELLS.

A striking change was found in the iodinated protein patterns
of three clones of NIL8 cells transformed by hamster sarcoma
virus (HSV) (Fig. 3 b, c, d) and two clones of NIL clone 1 transformed by polyoma virus (Fig. 3 g and h). In the case of the HSV-
transformed cells the major iodinated band (band 1) was missing
and in the polyoma transformed cells it was greatly reduced. The
change in the transformed cells is confined to a reduction or loss
of band 1 and the other labelled proteins seem to be unaffected.

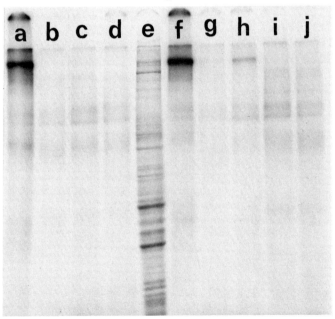

Fig. 3.   Iodination of normal and virus-transformed NIL
cells.   Autoradiogram of 7. 5% gel.   (a) NIL8; (b) NIL8-HSV6;
(c) NIL8-HSV9; (d) NIL8-HSV11; (e) NIL8 labelled with ^{14}C-
leucine; (f) NIL clone 1 (g) NIL clone 1-Py1; (h) NIL clone 1-Py8;
(i) NIL clone 1-HSV1; (j) NIL clone 1-HSV3.   Iodinated samples
contained equal amounts of protein.

In chicken embryo fibroblasts transformed by a mutant of Rous sarcoma virus which is temperature sensitive for the induction of the transformed phenotype the band 1 protein was much reduced in cells at the permissive temperature compared with cells shifted to the non-permissive temperature.

There are several possible explanations for the loss of band 1 protein in the transformed cells viz. 1) it is not made or is made in reduced amounts. 2) it is synthesized at the same rate as in untransformed cells but is (a) masked from the iodination procedure, (b) is promptly degraded or (c) turns over rapidly. Since transformed cells metabolically labelled with sugars do not have a band corresponding to band 1 (Fig. 2 c, i) cells, it is unlikely that it is masked. The possibility that the protein is incomplete or modified in transformed cells cannot be assessed until it has been more completely characterised chemically, serologically or biologically.

The possibility that band 1 is synthesized but lost by proteolytic degradation would be in accord with the observation that it is very susceptible to tryptic digestion (Fig. 4). Also transformed cells have been shown in a number of cases to have greater proteolytic activity than their untransformed precursors (6, 7).

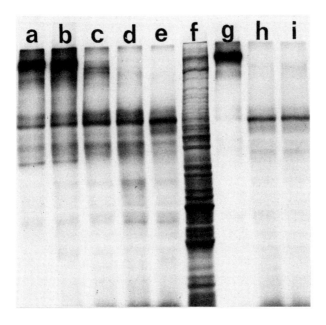

Fig. 4. The effect of tryptic digestion on the pattern of iodination of NIL8 cells. Autoradiogram of 7.5% gel (a-e) NIL8 cells
iodinated and subsequently treated before harvest with : (a) 10μg/
ml trypsin + 10μg/ml Soyabean trypsin inhibitor for 10 min. (b)
1μg/ml trypsin for 1 min (c) 1μg/ml trypsin for 5 min (d) 1μg/ml
trypsin for 10 min; (e) 10μg/ml trypsin for 10 min. All at room
temperature in phosphate buffered saline pH 7.3; (f) C-leucine
labelled NIL8 cells; (g) cells iodinated and harvested without
further treatment; (h) and (i) cells treated with trypsin (10μg/ml
for 10 min) before, (h) or after (i), iodination. Iodinated samples
comprised equal amounts of radioactivity.

Of particular interest in this respect are the recent studies by Reich and his colleagues (8, 9, 10) which have shown that transformed cells generate proteolytic activity in culture by producing a factor which activates serum plasminogen to plasmin. They have also shown that transformed cells cultured in medium prepared with plasminogen-free serum fail to express some of their transformed properties.

These observations suggest a number of obvious experiments which may bring about the reappearance of band 1 in transformed cells. However the treatment of NIL8-HSV cells with a variety of protease inhibitors have so far failed to lead to the expression of band 1 in these cells or cause a reversion of transformed morphology.

Some indication that the transformed cells have the ability to degrade band 1 protein comes from an experiment in which a culture of iodinated NIL8 cells lost their band 1 protein after co-cultivation with an equal number of NIL8-HSV cells for 24 hrs.

THE BIOLOGICAL SIGNIFICANCE OF THE CELL SURFACE PROTEINS

The major surface protein of normal cells which is depleted or missing in transformed cells is removed by the same degree of mild tryptic digestion that in some cell systems stimulates quiescent cells to undergo a further round of cell division (11, 12) and also renders these cells agglutinable by the same reduced concentration of lectins effective on their transformed derivatives (12).

Some of the properties of transformed cells seem to be associated with their inability to be checked in a non-growing post-mitotic phase. e. g. the completion of the carbohydrate moiety of certain normal cell glycolipids seems to take place at the cell growth "bottleneck" in the early part of the G1 phase (13) and the loss of this synthetic capacity in transformed cells may be directly associated with their free passage from mitosis to the S period and on to the next cell division. The possibility that a similar situation holds for the synthesis of band 1 protein cannot be definitely answered at present. It has been found however that as the density of NIL8 cultures increases, the amount of band 1 available for iodination at the cell surface increases (Fig. 5).

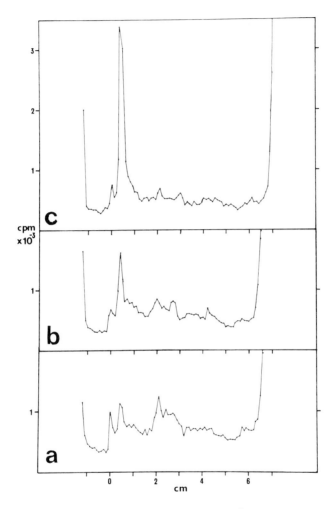

Fig. 5. SDS- polyacrylamide gels of NIL8 cells iodinated at different densities. Replicate cultures were iodinated on successive days when; a) subconfluent, exponentially growing; b) about confluent but still some mitoses; c) confluent, no mitoses. Equal amounts of protein were applied in each case to cylindrical gels which were cut into 1mm slices after electrophoresis. Gels were 7.5% with 5% stacking gel. Electrophoresis from left to right. 0cm represents interface between stacking and running gels.

This is consistent with the maximum expression of the protein occurring at the stage of normal cell inhibition in G1. When NIL8 cells are held at the G1/S interphase by hydroxyurea inhibition the amount of band 1 is not increased relative to exponentially growing cells. This indicates that cessation of growth per se is insufficient to cause the accumulation of band 1 protein. Sparse cells blocked in low serum medium resemble dense quiescent cells in their content of band 1. A similar response to inhibitors was found for the "density dependent" glycosphingolipids (13). Also cells arrested in colchicine-induced metaphase express very little if any band 1. Given these facts it is tempting to indulge in the luxury of speculation about possible roles for band 1 proteins as a regulator of cell growth. It is conceivable that the accumulation of such a protein to a critical concentration in the plasma membrane could affect a number of functions e.g. by masking receptor groups, competing for growth activators, blocking transport systems or affecting the fluidity of the membrane. We are at present studying some of these possibilities.

REFERENCES

1.   R.O. Hynes, Proc. Nat. Acad. Sci. U.S., 70 (1973) 3170.

2.   L. Diamond, Int. J. Cancer, 2 (1967) 143.

3.   J. Zavada and I. Macpherson, Nature, 225 (1970) 24.

4.   J. Graham, Biochem. J. 130 (1972) 1113.

5.   R.O. Hynes and K.C. Humphryes, J. Cell Biol., in press.

6.   H.B. Bosmann, Biochim. Biophys. Acta 264 (1972) 339.

7.   H.P. Schnebli, Schweiz. Med. Wochenschr., 102 (1972) 1194.

8.   J.C. Unkeless, A. Tobia, L. Ossowski, J.P. Quigley, D.B. Rifkin, and E. Reich, J. Exp. Med. 137 (1973) 85.

9.   L. Ossowski, J.C. Unkeless, A. Tobia, J.P. Quigley, D.B. Rifkin and E. Reich, J. Exp. Med. 137 (1973) 112.

10.   L. Ossowski, J.P. Quigley, G.M. Kellerman and E. Reich, J. Exp. Med., 138 (1973) 1056.

11.   B. M. Sefton and H. Rubin, Nature, 227, (1970) 843.

12.   M. M. Burger, Nature, 227 (1970) 170.

13.   D. R. Critchley, K. A. Chandrabose, J. M. Graham and
      I. Macpherson, in: Control of proliferation in animal
      cells. eds. B. Clarkson and R. Baserga. Cold Spring
      Harbor Press. in press.

DISCUSSION

M. J. Weber, University of Illinois: I was interested in your remark that addition of protease inhibitors didn't restore the band one protein to transformed cells and I was wondering whether you had monitored any other aspects of the transformed phenotype to see if the protease inhibitor would restore those to normal, under your conditions.

I. MacPherson, Imperial Cancer Research Fund Laboratories: Yes, we have studied a number of protease-inhibitors, eg. soybean trypsin inhibitor, ovomucoid, TLCK etc. We did not obtain results comparable to those published by Schnebli and Burger who found that protease-inhibitors caused a slowing of transformed 3T3 growth. They suggest that these cells may, like normal cells, be blocked in the G1 phase. Some of these protein inhibitors (eg. TLCK) are quite toxic and may simply slow down the cell metabolism. What may appear to be a cell that has been regulated or blocked may just be rather sick.

M. J. Weber: Well, we have found that addition of TLCK to Rous-transformed chick cells can return the high rate of hexose transport found in those cells to the normal level and can increase cellular adhesiveness (both of which are cell surface properties) and can also restore morphology to normal. I presented the data yesterday but thought that I would mention it again because so many people were watching the alligators. It is true that the protease inhibitors are very toxic and it is important to monitor the cell culture conditions very carefully to get them to work properly, rather than just killing the cells. If you add TLCK to cultures that are too sparce or if you add it to freshly seeded cultures, then the cells are very much more sensitive to the toxic effects of the inhibitors. The toxic dose and the effective dose of TLCK are very close, so it seems to me that, in this case, the negative result is not as significant as the positive result. I also would like to ask another question. You demonstrated the growth state dependence of the synthesis of the band one protein and I was wondering if you have looked for it in confluent but rapidly growing cells--for example cells that have been fluid changed to fresh medium on a daily or twice daily basis.

I. MacPherson: When NIL8 cells reach confluence they slow down considerably, even with frequent medium changes.

M. J. Weber: Well I am asking because Wickus & Ribbins have been looking at the synthesis of a similar protein and the way they keep their cells growing is by frequent medium changes, even past confluence. I am wondering whether or not the appearance of the band one protein in normal cells might in some way be associated with contact between cells irrespective of the growth rate of the cell.

I. MacPherson: Well the short answer to these questions is no we haven't done them, but I can say the synthesis, or rather the expression of this protein increases significantly as the culture increases in density and the cells make contact. However, it may be possible to distinguish between contact and the depletion of serum growth promoters in the way you suggest.

G. Koch, Roche Institute of Molecular Biology: I have a short comment with regard to the use of protease inhibitors in cell cultures. Pong in my laboratory has recently observed that the trypsin inhibitor TPCK specifically inhibits initiation of protein synthesis.

M. Lubin, Dartmouth Medical School: Does dibutyryl cyclic AMP induce an iodinatable special band in your system or that of any other laboratory?

I. MacPherson: This is being studied at present but we do not yet have any substantial data.

M. Lubin: And a second short question in anticipation of tommorrow's talk. What is the pH optimum for inducing this band?

I. MacPherson: With apologies to Dr. Eagle - we have not done these experiments.

M. Rieber, Rutgers University: With regard to the clear differences you have observed between normal and transformed cells and growing cells and resting cells. Have you done the experiment in which you prelabel the cells and follow the fate of the iodinated tyrosine in the cases where you see it disappear from that iodinated peak.

I. MacPherson: Well we have experimented with a TS/RSV mutant in chick embryo cells and it will take too long to go into detail. However, the protein is lost in a temperature down shift, that is from the non-permissive to the permissive temperature and reappears in the shift to non-permissive temperature but the change in both cases is unexpectedly slow.

W.S. Lynn, Duke Medical Center: Do you have any evidence that these cells, any of these clones do make tryptic inhibitors and if so, what is their rate of turn-over, etc?

I. MacPherson: Do you mean the normal clones?

W.S. Lynn: Well, the various clones which you are playing with. Is their any evidence that any of these cells make tryptic inhibitors or protease inhibitors of any type.

I. MacPherson: Do you mean, could we induce the reappearance of band 1 protein in transformed cells? Is that what you had in mind?

W.S. Lynn: No, I am asking if any of these cells do produce any proteolytic inhibitors?

I. MacPherson: We have no evidence to suggest that.

P.A. Srere, Veterans Administration Hospital: Have you had a chance to compare a suspension grown cell line with the same cell line grown on monolayers?

I. MacPherson: We haven't done that.

H. Eagle, Albert Einstein College of Medicine: Dr. MacPherson, you have shown virus transformation causes the disappearance of band one. Do you see the appearance of a new protein, perhaps associated with Dr. Warren's carbohydrate peak A?

I. MacPherson: It would not show up in the technique we used. His glycopeptides are removed from the surface of the cells by trypsinization and then treated with pronase, so it becomes a small glycopeptide. It would not show on our gels.

S. Sorof, Institute of Cancer Research: Have you examined whether or not the proteins of band 1 are present in cells growing in plasminogen-depleted medium?

I. MacPherson: Yes, we have done some experiments to study this but the results are unclear. From the work of Dr. Reich and his colleagues, it seems that the species of the serum relative to the species of the cell is very important. We have tried the appropriate serum and cell combinations and we did try to make plasminogen-free serum but the results were inconclusive. We have received some kosher plasminogen-free serum from Dr. Riech and we will do experiments with that.

S. Roseman, Johns Hopkins University: I don't think enough attention has been paid at this meeting to the microexudate which cells put out and which is on the bottom of the dish. I should imagine that this material would be of particular interest or concern to you. Are you sealing with microexudates in other words?

I. MacPherson: Does the microexudate come off the surface with versene?

S. Roseman: I don't know whether anybody has really defined it except that it is there.

I. MacPherson: Well you get the same results if the cells are scraped off or the cells are removed in versene.

Perhaps you can make something out of that.

S. Roseman: OK, I don't know what makes the micro-exudate stick to the glass, but possibly it is ionic bonds, in which case perhaps EDTA might take it off.

GROWTH BEHAVIOR OF TRANSFORMED CELLS AS RELATED TO THE SURFACE STRUCTURES OF GLYCOLIPIDS AND GLYCOPROTEINS

S.HAKOMORI, C.G.GAHMBERG, R.A.LAINE AND D.KIEHN
Department of Pathobiology
School of Public Health and Department of Microbiology
School of Medicine, University of Washington, Seattle

Abstract: Tumor cells have been characterized by the following phenotypes expressed on cell surface membranes:

1) Defective synthesis of glycolipids resulting in a reduced concentration/or absence of a certain glycolipid. This was occasionally accompanied by an accumulation of its precursor glycolipid.

2) Absence of a high molecular"galactoprotein a", irrespective of cell contact. The label of this protein in normal NIL cells increased greatly at confluent phase and was absent in trypsinized cells.

3) Increase of a particular sialylgalacto/or galactosaminoprotein in NILpy, 3T3sv, and 3T3svpy cells These glycoproteins are absent in the confluent phase of normal NIL and 3T3 cells, but detectable in growing cells, and were greatly increased in transformed cells.

4) The label in glycolipids increased in G_1 and decreased in mitotic phase, showing an obvious dependency on the cell cycle of NIL cells. Presence of a glycolipid label characteristic to transformed NILpy cells was detected.

The change of growth behavior induced by cyclic AMP, galactose, and by dextran sulfate greatly altered the surface glycoprotein and glycolipid profile determined by external glycosyl labeling.

These changes were discussed in view of growth control changes through surface modifications by anti-glycolipid antibodies and by glycolipid enrichment in membranes.

INTRODUCTION

Transformed cells have been characterized by the change of phenotypes expressed in membrane functions, especially those of surface membranes (see 1). Major focuses in studying such aberrant phenotypes of tumor cells in this laboratory have been: 1) change of chemical structure and components of glycosphingolipids; and 2) organizational status of membrane glycolipids and glycoproteins revealed by the surface labeling procedure and by reactivities of cells to specific antibodies directed against glycosphingolipids.

The change of glycolipid compositions associated with chemical or viral transformation of cells has been increasingly apparent since the first demonstration of hematoside decrese and lactosylceramide increase in transformed "BHK" cells (2). Recent studies on fucolipid changes in various fibroblastic cells transformed by oncornaviruses (3) and of ganglioside changes in chemically induced solid mammary tumors in vivo (4) are particularly noticeable. Due to blocked glycosyltransferases, and by loss of "glycosyl extension" on cell contact (5), many transformed cells have been characterized by defective synthesis of higher glycolipids. The blocked synthesis can be seen in GM_2-ganglioside (6,7), hematoside (8), ceramide trihexoside (9), disialoganglioside (4), and in blood group A and B glycosphingolipids (10).

Since the topics dealing with defective synthesis of glycolipids and cell contact-dependent change of glyco-lipid composition have been extensively reviewed elsewhere (11,12), this paper will give only a very brief description focusing on recent developments in blocked synthesis of blood group glycolipids. The major part of this paper will deal with recent studies carried out in this laboratory regarding the alteration of surface glycoprotein and glyco-lipids detected by the surface labeling procedure.

EXPERIMENTAL

Characterization of glycolipids and determination of enzymatic activities for glycolipid synthesis: Glyco-lipids were separated by the acetylation procedure (13), and characterized by enzymatic hydrolysis and chemical determination of components. In some cases, methylation has been applied in order to obtain positional information of linkages. Typical examples have been described in a series of papers on characterization of globoside (14), cytolipin R (15, 15a), blood group H (16), and A (17) glycolipids.

Enzymatic synthesis of glycolipid was determined by incubation of radioactive sugar nucleotide and substrate glycolipids dissolved in buffers without interaction with metals and phosphate, containing non-ionic detergents according to the methods described by Basu, Kaufman, and Roseman (18) and by Hildebrand and Hauser (19). Preparation of active transferases with higher activities was achieved by brief sonication rather than Potter homogenization (9).

The activities of synthetases were expressed by the yield of radioactive incorporation into glycolipid product as catalyzed by 1 mg of protein per one hour. Radioactive glycolipid products were usually extensively characterized chemically, immunologically, and enzymatically as described previously (9,10).

Cells: Mouse 3T3 cells, 3T6 and 3T3 transformed with Simian virus 40 (3T3sv) and double transformed with Simian virus 40 and polyoma virus (3T3svpy) were cultured in Dulbecco-modified Eagle's medium (in 5% CO_2 atmosphere). Hamster NIL and BHK cells were grown in Eagle's medium in 3% CO_2 atmosphere. Transformed cells changed their morphology and became sensitive to contact inhibition of growth when cultured in original Eagle's medium with one times amino acids and vitamins and 10% calf serum, containing/ml 10 µg (for 3T6 cells) or 4 µg (for NILpy) of dextran sulfate (20). The dextran sulfate (m.w. 50,000) was donated by Dr. Goto, Tohoku University, Sendai, Japan. With increased amino acids, vitamins, and fetal calf serum, the changes of morphology and contact sensitivity were $1-1.5\times10^5/cm^2$, respectively. Cell growth was not stimulated by change of medium containing dextran sulfate at the confluent phase. Cells grown in regular medium reached densities as high as $10^6/cm^2 -- 3\times10^6/cm^2$.

NILpy and 3T3svpy cells were grown in the presence of 0.1 mM dibutyryl cyclic AMP and 1 mM of theophyllin according to the method described by Sheppard (21). The morphology of NILpy cells appeared to change more remarkably than that of 3T3svpy cells. After 2-3 days in culture,

the cells appeared well contact-oriented and their sizes
increased. Freshly transformed NILpy cells showed remarkable changes in morphology and contact orientation when
cultured in Eagle's medium (two times amino acids and
vitamins), in which glucose was replaced with galactose
and supplemented with 10% fetal calf serum (22).

Surface labeling: The procedure for surface labeling
was a slight modification of a method previously described
(23, 24). The cells from one plate (Falcon, 14 cm diameter)
were enough for labeling, and were obtained either by
scraping with a rubber policeman or by using a 0.02% EDTA
solution or a 0.25% trypsin solution (Grant Island Biological Company). The cells were washed twice by centrifugation in phosphate-buffered saline PH 7.0. 0.5 ml PBS was
added, containing 2mM phenylmethlysulfonylfluoride (Sigma)
to inhibit proteases. 100 µl galactose oxidase dissolved
in PBS pH 7.0 containing 100 units per ml (Sigma Type III)
was then added, and the cells were incubated at room temperature for two hours with gentle shaking. In some experiments, galactose oxidase solution was placed on cells
grown in plastic plates after cell sheets were washed with
phosphate buffered saline pH 7.0. After two hours' incubation, cells were separated by EDTA and then treated with
(^{3}H) sodium borohydride after washing with PBS pH 7.4 (see
below). The galactose oxidase preparation contained no
measurable proteolytic or neuraminidase a tivity. In some
experiments, galactose oxidase was purified by affinity
chromatography; namely, the enzyme was specifically
absorbed on a column of "Sepharose 4B" (Pharmacia Fine
Chemical, through Sigma Chemical Company) at 4° and eluted
with 10% galactose. The enzyme, obtained after dialysis
of the eluate, was freed from impurities as judged by gel
electrophoresis. After incubation the cells were washed
twice in PBS pH 7.4. The cell pellet was suspended in 0.5
ml of PBS pH 7.4 to which was added 50 µl of tritiated
sodium borohydride solution containing 0.5-1 mCi NaB^{3}H$_4$,
specific activity 6 Ci/mM (new England Nuclear). The
reaction mixture was allowed to stand for 30 minutes at
room temperature. In some experiments the cells were first
incubated with 50 µl <u>Vibrio cholerae</u> neuraminidase (Calbiochem, Type B containing 500 units per ml) in 0.5 ml 0.1
M phosphate buffer pH 6.0. Cells incubated with dibutyryl
cyclic AMP were treated with neuraminidase in the presence
of 1 mM concentration of dibutyryl cyclic AMP and followed

by the labeling procedure.

Analysis of labeled glycoproteins and glycolipids:
The labeled cells were dissolved in an aqueous solution
containing 1% of sodium dodecyl sulfate with 5% of 2-mercap-
toethanol by heating at 100° for two minutes. β-galacto-
sidase (m.w. 136,000), bovine serum albumin (m.w. 68,000),
ovalbumin (m.w. 44,500), and cytochrome C (m.w. 11,700),
labeled respectively by ^{14}C-formaldehyde (25), were added
as internal markers. Electrophoresis was carried out and
the radioactive gels sliced and counted as described
previously (26). Unless otherwise indicated, the cells
were harvested with 0.02% EDTA treatment.

Glycolipids were extracted and partitioned according to
Folch et al (26). The neutral glycolipid fraction was
purified from the lower phase by the acetylation procedure
(24), and analyzed by thin-layer chromatography on Silica
gel G with the solvent mixture chloroform-methanol-water
(65:30:8); the following glycolipids were co-chromato-
graphed: globoside, Forssman glycolipid, ceramide trihexoside, and ceramide lactoside. The radioactivity of
each glycolipid was determined after the bands were scraped
and treated with "NCS" solubilizer (Amersham/Searle).
Total radioactivities were determined after NCS solubilization of cell aliquots and counted in a toluene-based scintillation fluid. The labeled glycolipid was extracted
from thin-layer plate after they were separated, and
determined carbohydrate components by gas-chromatography
after methanolysis and trimethylsilylation (27). Radioactivities of each peak were determined as previously
described (23).

RESULTS

1. *Deficient synthesis of glycolipids with accumulation
of precursor glycolipids.*

Glycolipid composition has been compared between a
number of normal and transformed cells, including those of
transformed cells by temperature sensitive mutants of
tumor viruses. Comparison was also made between normal
and chemically transformed cells in vitro including various human tumor tissues. Without exception, glycolipid
patterns of tumors were found to be profoundly different
from normal cells or tissues (see for review; ref. 11,12).

Deficient synthesis of glycolipids with simultaneous accumulation of precursor glycolipid has been the major change. Depending on the types of cells studied or transforming agents applied, we observed block of enzyme activities related to glycolipid synthesis can be greatly varied. Defective synthesis of ganglioside and neutral glycolipid due to blocked glycosyl transferase activities has been found in various laboratories listed in Table 1. As mentioned in the "Introduction," this block of glycolipid synthesis could be a common denominator of transformed phenotype.

In human adenocarcinoma, a deletion of blood groups A and B determinants with accumulation of H or Lewis antigens has been reported (28). This suggests that synthesis of A or B determinants could be blocked in human adenocarcinoma. Consequently, synthesis of A^a-glycolipid (17) from H_1-glycolipid (16) has been compared between the enzyme fraction of human gastrointestinal mucosa and that of human gastrointestinal adenocarcinoma. Figure 1 shows one example of the difference in A^a-glycolipid synthesis from H_1-glycolipid demonstrated by enzyme fraction ("p-2+3") derived from normal gastric mucosa and that of gastric cancer.

On the other hand, it is interesting to note that those enzymes which were "blocked" in transformed cells showed contact-dependent enhancement in non-transformed progenitor cells (see Table 2). It was interpreted, therefore, that enzyme block for synthesis of higher glycolipid could be ascribed to a deficient glycosylation of transformed cells on cell contact.

Further studies on glycolipid of BHK cells and BHK transformed by "ts-3 mutants" showed that glycosylation on cell to cell contact does not occur in the same molecule that shows deficient synthesis in a transformed state (29; and Gahmberg, Kiehn, and Hakomori, 34). These two phenomena, *i.e.*, contact dependent glycolipid changes and transformation-dependent glycolipid changes are not always related. They are probably controled under independent mechanisms (34).

TABLE 1

Block of glycolipid: glycosyltransferases in various transformed cells

Block of enzyme reaction	Cells	References
Gal1→4Glc→Cer+UDPGalNAc ⟶ ↑ Sial GalNAc→Gal1→4Glc→ceramide ↑ Sial	3T3sv AL/Nsv 3T3mlv	Cumar et al (6) Mora et al (7)
Gal1→4Glc→Cer+CMP-Sial ⟶ Sial2→3Gal1→4Glc→ceramide	BHKpy	Den et al (8)
Gal1→4Glc→Cer+UDPGal ⟶ Galα1→4Galβ1→4Glc→Cer	BHKpy NILpy	Kijimoto & Hakomori (9)
Gal1→3GalNAc1→4Gal→Glc→ceramide ↑ Sial + CMP-Sial ⟶ Gal→GalNAc1→4Gal→Glc→Cer ↑ ↑ Sial Sial	Mammary cancer induced by benzan-thracene	Keenan & Morré (4)
Fuc1→2Galβ1→4GlcNAcβ1→3Gal1→4Glc→Cer +UDP-GalNAc ⟶ Fuc1→2Galβ1→4GlcNAcβ1→3Gal1→4Glc→Cer ↑ GalNAc	Human adeno-carcinoma	Stellner & Hakomori (10)

sv: transformed cells carrying Simian virus 40
py: transformed cells carrying polyoma virus
mlv: murine leukemia virus

TABLE 2

Enhancement of UDP-Galactose:lactosylceramideɑ-Galactosyl-
transferase activity in NIL cells on increased cell population density and defect of such enzyme response in polyoma
transformed NIL cells (from Kijimoto and Hakomori, Biochem.
Biophys. Res. Commun. 44, 557, 1971)

| Cells | Population density per cm^2 | Glycolipid synthesized in μμmoles/mg P-3 protein */per hour (complete systems†) | |
| | | Activities of enzymes | |
		Galβ→Glc→Cer+UDPGal →Galɑ→Galβ→Glc→Cer	Glc→Cer+UDPGal→ Galβ→Glc→Cer
NIL	Sparse	$\leq 5 \times 10^4$	385	247
	Confluent	$> 10^5$	1052	257
NILpy	Sparse	$\leq 10^5$	26	400
	High	$> 10^5$	38	206

*Cells briefly sonicated (60 watts; 90 sec); centrifuged
800xg 15 minutes; the supernatant centrifuged in a Sorvall
12,000xg 25 minutes; the supernatant was centrifuged in a
Spinco at 105,000xg for one hour; the precipitate was
assigned as "P-3."

†0.05 μ mole of substrate lipid; 800 μg "Cutscum"; 10 μl
1M cacodylate buffer pH 6.1; 20 μl 0.15 M $MnCl_2$; 20 μl
of (14_C)-UDP-Gal which contained 1.4×10^5 cmp/80 mμ moles.

Fig. 1. *Example of blocked synthesis of glycolipid in tumor compared to normal tissue (from Stellner and Hakomori, Biochemical Biophysical Research Communication 55, 439-445, 1973).*

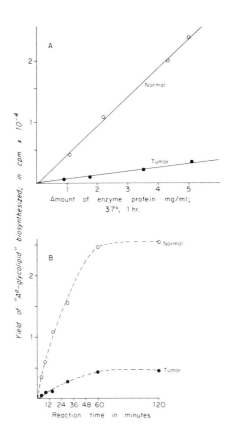

The difference of reactivities depending on the amount of enzyme protein (A) and on the reaction time (B). The quantity of enzyme protein used in experiment B was 5 mg/ml (300 µg/100 µl). Open circle: normal gastric mucosal epithelia; solid circle: tumor. The reaction is essentially due to enzyme activity which catalyzes conversion of H_1 glycolipid to A^a-glycolipid.

2. The presence of a high molecular "galactoprotein a" in confluent cells, absence of this label in growing or tryp-sinized and in transformed cells.

Hamster fibroblasts either NIL or BHK cells showed a surface galactoprotein label with approximate molecular weight 200,000. The label of this protein was most remarkable at complete confluency but disappeared almost completely in polyoma transformed cells (Fig. 2). Growing cells (at the logarithmic phase) showed a very small quantity of this label and greatly increased when cell growth ceased at confluency. The label completely dis-appeared on trypsinization (34).

The label of "galactoprotein a" was followed immediate-ly after the confluent NIL cells were typsinized. The intensity of this label appeared at G_1 phase, persistent during S and M-phase. The label in glycolipid showed an obvious dependency on cell cycle as seen in Fig. 3.

A glycoprotein similar to "galactoprotein a" was also found in BHK C13/21 cells at the confluent phase, which disappeared on trypsinization and in malignant transform-ants by polyoma virus. The presence of this galacto-protein at the confluent phase appears to be correlated with polyoma gene expression as it appeared at permissive temperature of ts-3-transformed BHK cells (BHKpy-ts-3) and disappeared completely at non-permissive temperature (Gahmberg, Kiehn, and Hakomori, ref. 34).

3. The appearance of a new sialylgalactosyl/or galacto-saminyl label on surfaces of growing as well as transformed 3T3 and NIL cells.

a. <u>Mouse fibroblast 3T3 cells</u> show very little surface label when the galactose oxidase procedure is directly applied to intact cells; the label can be greatly increased after cells are treated with neuraminidase; thus the label for glycoprotein peaks a to f can be distinguished by acrylamide gel electrophoresis. All these peaks represent therefore sialylgalactosyl/or sialylgalactosaminyl pro-teins. A large lipid label L consists of an essentially non-specific label yet unidentified. Glycoprotein peaks are all specific except some of the label contained in peak e. The contact inhibited confluent 3T3 cells had no label at the peak c (Fig. 5-A) which appeared clearly at the growing stage (Fig. 5-B), as well as on cells after trypsin

78

treatment (Fig. 5-E). The peak c and non-specific peak e were treatly enhanced in 3T3sv cells (Fig. 5-C) or in 3T3svpy cells (Fig. 5-D).

b. NIL cells after neuraminidase treatment also showed a similar label as peak c of 3T3 cells, which increased significantly on NILpy cells as well as in trypsinized cells. (Fig. 5-F, G; "peak d"). The behavior of the sialylgalactosylglycoprotein represented by "peak c" of 3T3 cells or by "peak d" of NIL cells opposed to the behavior of a high molecular "galactoprotein a" as is described in the previous section. The activity of the label in those sialylglycoprotein is higher in growing cells, as well as in transformed cells; their label decreased and almost non-detectable when cells were confluent. This behavior resembled that of sialylglycopeptide described by Warren and his associates (32, 33).

4. *Changes of surface label of transformed cells (NILpy, 3T3sv, 3T3svpy) associated with the change of growth behavior (induced contact responses).*

Growth behaviors and contact responses (contact inhibitability and orientation) of transformed cells greatly altered when the transformed cells were cultured in the presence of cyclic AMP (35,36) galactose (22), and dextran sulfate (20).

In the culture medium in which glucose was replaced by galactose, NILpy cells showed a remarkable cell orientation and enhanced contact inhibitability (saturation cell density reduced) (22). The surface structures of such cells was characterized by a remarkable enhancement in the label of galactoprotein b and c. The label of globoside was also enhanced in NILpy cells when contact response was obviously enhanced as previously reported (24).

Both 3T3svpy cells and NILpy cells whose contact responses were greatly enhanced by culturing those cells in the presence of cyclic AMP and theophylin showed an enhanced label at peaks b and d (Fig. 6).

5. *Presence of a specific label in glycolipids of transformed cells (NILpy) and its absence in NIL cells.*

In a number of studies on glycolipid label, the presence of a specific label in terminal galactosyl residue of glycolipid was observed. Such a label was not detectable in NIL cells and therefore is considered a specific for

Fig. 2. *Surface galactosyl or galactosaminyl label in glycoproteins and glycolipids of intact NIL and NILpy cells*

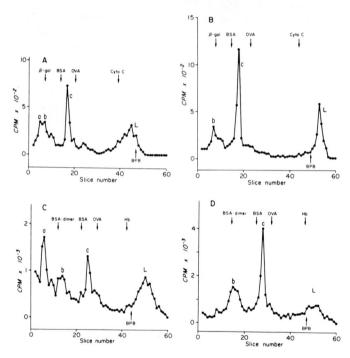

A and C: NIL confluent cells, B and D: NILpy cells. The pattern was obtained by sodium dodecyl sulfate-polyacrylamide gel electrophoresis run in 7.5% gel for A, B, and in 5% gel for C, D. Note the presence of peak a (referred to as "galactoprotein a" in the text) is only present in normal NIL cells and deleted in NILpy cells. This is a galactoprotein with molecular weight calculated as 200,000. Peak b is not greatly different between NIL and NILpy cells; peak c contains non-specific label i.e. labeled by tritiated sodium borohydride alone. Peak L contains glycolipid label and non-specific label. Chemical nature of non-specific label could be: fatty aldehyde (plasmal), ketosphingosine, proteins containing pyridinium nucleus (hemproteins), phosphoprotein containing acylphosphate bond (30), protein containing reducible Schiff base such as collageneous protein (31), etc.

Fig. 3. *Change of the surface label in glycolipids during cell cycle.*

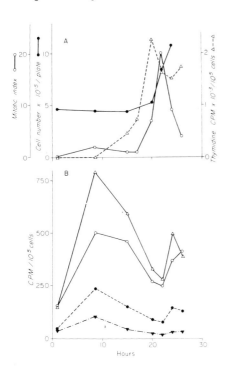

A: change of mitotic index (o—o—o), cell number (●—●—●), and thymidine uptake (Δ--Δ-Δ).

B: change of activity of glycolipids in cpm per 10^5 cells.

Forssman glycolipid (o- o- o), globoside (Δ- Δ -Δ), ceramide trihexoside (●--●--●), and ceramide dihexoside (▼—▼--▼). Note that activities in glycolipids enhance before the peak of thymidine uptake (S-phase).

Legend for Fig. 4 as shown on next page: Patterns A, B, C, D, E, and F were obtained from synchronized cell cultures corresponding to 1, 8.5, 15, 20, 22, and 24 hrs. after seeding of cells. Each point corresponds to the time shown in Fig. 3.

Fig. 4. *Surface glycoprotein label in NIL cells at different stages of cell cycle.*

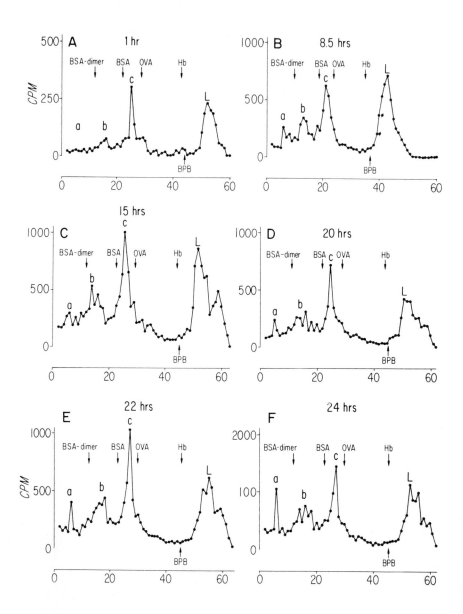

Fig.5 *Surface sialylgalactosyl/or sialygalactosaminyl label in 3T3 cells*

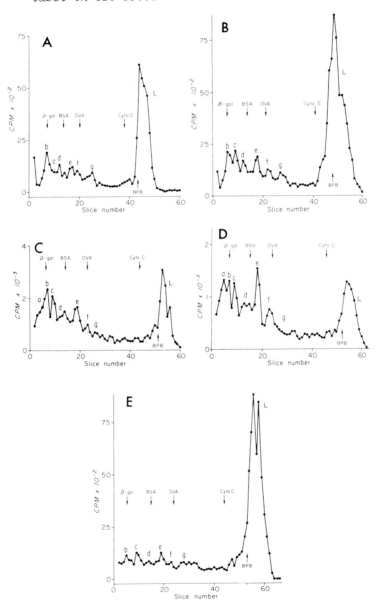

Fig. 5 continued . . *Surface sialylgalactosyl/or sialygalactosaminyl label in NIL cells*

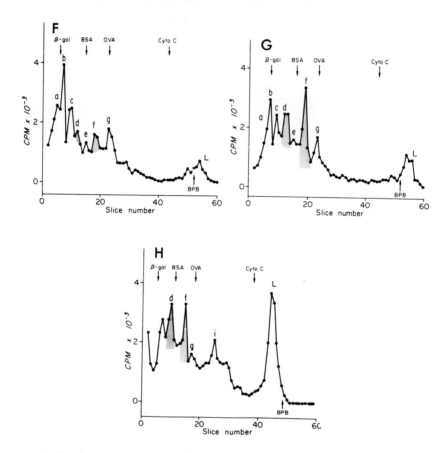

Cells harvested with 0.02% EDTA were incubated with 50 ul of Vibrio cholerae neureuminidase (Calbiochem, type B) that contained 500 units/ml in 0.5 ml of 0.1 M phosphate buffer pH 6.0 containing 2 mM phenylmethlysulfonylfluoride (Sigma), then process surface label with galactose oxidase and tritiated borohydride.

A confluent 3T3 cells; B growing sparse 3T3 cells; C 3T3 sv, D 3T3 svpy; E 3T3 cells trypsin treated; F confluent NIL; G NILpy cells; H NIL trypsin treated.

Fig. 6. *Surface sialylgalactosyl/or sialyl galacto-saminyl label in NILpy and 3T3sv cells when growth behavior of these cells was modified.*

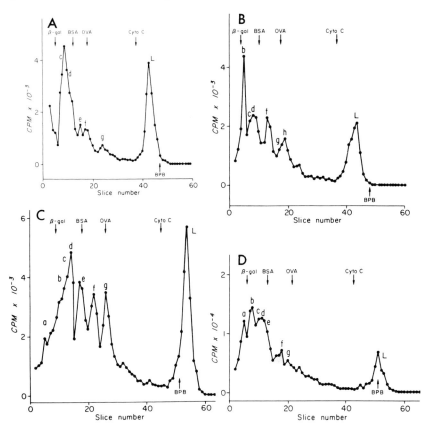

A: 3T3sv cells grown in medium containing cyclic AMP. B: NILpy cells grown in medium containing cyclic AMP. Morphology and orientation of these cells were noticed greatly changed. C: NILpy cells grown in medium in which glucose was replaced with galactose. D: NILpy cells grown in the presence of dextran sulfate.

transformed cells.

In NIL cells the label was found in galactosamine residue of Forssman glycolipid or in globoside which was separated by thin-layer chromatography, but the label in galactosyl residue of glycolipids migrating at the position between ceramide penta and tetrasaccharide was remarkable only in NILpy cells and was almost negligable in NIL cells. Chemical characterization of such a specific label for NILpy cells is now under active pursuit.

The activities of label in glycolipids of normal cells agree with the chemical quantities of glycolipids present in membranes, however the specific activities of some glycolipids in transformed cells were higher than those of normal cells. In NILpy cells the label in higher glycolipids (Forssman and globoside) increased when contact responses became conspicuous by either dextran sulfate, dibutyrylcyclic AMP, and by galactose (24).

DISCUSSION

Four types of surface label changes related to the change of growth behavior of cells have been observed: 1) cell cycle dependent changes, 2) cell contact dependent changes, 3) transformation dependent changes, and 4) changes dependent on growth behavior due to intracellular metabolic changes induced by cyclic AMP, galactose and dextran sulfate.

As is well demonstrated in NIL cells, the label in various neutral glycolipids with longer carbohydrate chains depends greatly on cell cycles (Fig. 3), whereas the label in "galactoprotein a" with molecular weight 200,000 depends on cell cycle but obvious change is due to cell contact. Although the same experiments were not done in BHK cells, the presence of "galactoprotein a" in confluent BHK cells obviously indicates that the label in this galactoprotein could be largely cell contact dependent. Cell contact dependent change of glycolipid synthesis has been described (5,9). A similar change of cell contact dependent increase of galactosyl residue has been detected with <u>Ricinus communis</u> lectin (37).

Complete absence of the label in "galactoprotein a" after typsin treatment and after viral transformation (NILpy or BHKpy), irrespective of the cell population densities, suggests strongly that cell contact dependent variation of either "exposure" or synthesis of "galacto-protein a" is not observed in transformed cells, i.e. either synthesis or organization of "galactoprotein a" seems to be defective in transformed cell surfaces. The change of the surface structure of transformed cells is persistently defective, irrespective of cell contact or on cycle, i.e. the frozen state of surface dynamicity. This figure is consistent with the observation that those transformed cells showed a defective synthesis in higher neutral glycolipids and in hematoside as described in the introduction.

Deficiency in "galactoprotein a" as well as in various glycolipids can be an expressed phenotype of malignancy, most probably linked to the action of viral genes in these transformed cells. However, as has been repeatedly demon-strated in various chemically transformed cells (4,38,39), deficient synthesis of glycolipids cannot be solely caused by action of viral genes.

The changes in surface label and in deficient synthesis of glycolipids related to viral gene action have been most directly verified by experiments using temperature sensi-tive mutants of RNA and DNA tumor viruses, i.e. 1) blocked synthesis of hematoside has been correlated to phenotypic expression of various strains of temperature sensitive mutants of Rous sarcoma virus in chick embryo fibroblasts (Hakomori and Vogt; unpublished observation); 2) the label in "galactoprotein a" and synthesis of hematoside and lactosylceramide have been correlated to the expression of polyoma ts-3 mutants in BHK cells (Gahmberg, Kiehn, and Hakomori, see ref. 34).

The surface labeling procedure cannot be applied to highly sialylated cells without pretreatment with siali-dase. Sialidase-treated cells have been shown to be labeled as characteristic pattern. Both 3T3 and NIL cells after treatment with sialidase, showed a very faint label at peak c (molecular weight 105,000) which was greatly enhanced by trypsin treatment. The same label was greatly enhanced in transformed 3T3 and NIL cells after neuramini-dase treatment. This peak represents sialosylgalactosyl residue. It is strongly suggested that the synthesis of such glycoprotein with definite molecular weight greatly increased in transformed as well as in growing cells. It is interesting to recall Warren's work that the synthesis of a specific sialylglycoprotein enhances greatly in transformed cells (32,33,43).

The label in glycolipids is rather complex and sometimes difficult to evaluate because of the presence of heavy "non-specific label" in lipid fraction which has not been fully identified. It is necessary, therefore, that each glycolipid be isolated by acetylation procedures (13) followed by separation on thin-layer chromatography and determination of the activities of sugars after methanolysis and gas-chromatography as trimethylsilyl derivatives (27). Activities of sugars in glycolipids with longer carbohydrate chains such as ceramide tetrasaccharide and ceramide pentasaccharides may well be dependent on the chemical quantities present in cells; however, those glycolipids with shorter carbohydrate chains, especially ceramide dihexoside (lactosylceramide) and galactosylceramide, was not labeled or was very weakly labeled. Nevertheless, relative increase of the label in ceramide trisaccharide or in disaccharide was observed in transformed NIL (NILpy) cells as previously reported (24).

The chemical quantities of ceramide tetrasaccharide (globoside) and of ceramide pentasaccharide (Forssman glycolipid) in NILpy cells were extremely low compared to progenitor NIL cells, nevertheless some labeled activities were still observed, i.e. specific activities of these glycolipids in transformed cells should be extremely high compared to the specific activities of those glycolipids in normal NIL cells. Among those glycolipids the presence of a new type of labeled galactosyl glycolipid with unknown chemical composition and structure was discovered, it may be specific for the transformed cells.

Information on cell surface glycoproteins and glycolipids of NILpy cells in contrast to NIL cells can be summarized as follows: 1) lack of "galactoprotein a," probably due to absence of cell contact dependent synthesis of this protein, 2) defective synthesis of globoside and Forssman glycolipid whose specific activities by surface label become relatively higher than normal NIL cells, 3) increase of a particular sialylgalactosylprotein "peak c," 4) presence of a new type of glycolipid characteristic to NILpy cells.

Other cells have not been as extensively studied as NIL and NILpy cells, but all or part of these changes could probably be found as well. Transformed 3T3 cells have been characterized by the phenomena 2) as previously described and defective synthesis of higher ganglioside has been reported previously (6,38,39,40).

As to the surface label changes occurring when the cellular metabolic patterns were changed, relatively little can be commented upon at the moment. Significantly, however, the surface organization/or synthesis of glyco-lipids and glycoproteins were greatly affected by the changes of intracellular metabolism induced by culturing cells in galactose medium or by the addition of metabolic regulator such as cyclic AMP.

Cells grown in galactose-replaced medium showed a greatly increased label in the galactoprotein b-c area when those cells exhibit obvious change of contact orientation. The surface changes may not happen immediate-ly after glucose in medium was replaced by galactose. As has been well illustrated by Kalckar and his associates (22), UDP-galactose, galactose-1-phosphate, and galactitol were accumulated due to UDP-galactose "epimerase choke" of NILpy cells. The metabolic pattern of galactose in those transformed cells showing "epimerase choke" could be partially normalized by culturing galactose medium, whereby an obvious change of surface structure was noticed. Through the change of surface galactoprotein, growth behavior can be affected by the altered intercellular recognition.

The effect of cyclic AMP on the surface glycoprotein label could be understood in the same way as the effect of galactose. In contrast to present study, previous works by Sakiyama and Robbins (42) and Yogeeswaran et al (40) showed that cyclic AMP did not affect the glycolipid pattern. Obvious changes of surface label pattern shown in this study clearly indicate that surface label is much more sensitive criteria than simple analysis of glycolipid level in picking up surface structures of cells indicative of growth behavior. Cyclic AMP may change intracellular metabolic patterns and consequently change the surface structure which determines growth behavior of cells.

All of these studies with surface labelling strongly suggest that social behavior of cells is determined by the presence or absence of specific glycoprotein or glycolipids, constituting surface structures through which cells can recognize each other. Another possibility is that glyco-proteins or glycolipids may assist transport of nutrients through cell surfaces or may regulate the fluid dynamic st-ate of plasma membranes.

If surface glycoproteins or glycolipids of membranes could be specifically modified or affected under physiolog-ical conditions, any effects on cell physiology and cell social behavior would be of great importance for establishi-ng direct relationship between cell surface structure and growth behavior of cells. This line of work has been act-ively pursued in our laboratory. Alpha-galactosidase and ficin can stimulate cell growth of NIL and BHK cells (un-published observation) this was considered analogous to the finding of Vaheri et al.that sialidase can stimulate growth of "contact inhibited cells" (44).

A most promising approach for specific modification of cell surface glycans has been investigated recently,namely:
1) Alteration of glycolipid composition in plasma mem-brane by exogenous addition of glycosphingolipid micelles in the cell growth medium.
2) Effect of purified antibodies against glycosphingo-lipids or their monovalent derivatives on the cell growth behavior and metabolism.

The former approach is based on the observation that glycosphinglipid antigens are readily taken up by cells to alter their immunologic specificities (45). In our preli-minary studies globoside added in culture medium was taken up by NIL cells and accumulate as a component of plasma membrane. This was evidenced by the recovery of ^{3}H-labeled globoside found in NIL cells cultured in medium containing globoside. NIL cells cultured in globoside-enriched medium (8 x 10^{-4} M globoside) reached 27 n moles per 10 mg cell residue in contrast to 12 n moles found in the same amount of cell residue from cells grown in normal medium.

Globoside enriched cells show the following changes in growth behavior :1) reduction of growth rate due to extended pre-replicative phase, and 2) a reduced cell saturation density which may result from changes in adhesive properties of cells (Laine and Hakomori,46). Extensive additional studies are necessary to determine the mechanism and specificities of this effect on cell growth.

The latter approach is only possible if antiglycolipid antibodies (47) were extensively purified by affinity column in which various glycosphingolipids were covalently linked to a substratum. The method for preparation of such affinity column is now established in this laboratory (Laine and Hakomori,48; Laine,Yogeeswaran, and Hakomori,49). The outline of the methods for preparation of neutral glycosphingolipids and gangliosides for attachement on solid substrates is shown in Figures 7 and 8. With these affinity columns, specific antibodies against neutral glycolipids and gangliosides can be purified extensively. It is noteworthy that the specificity of antihematoside isdirected to sialyl residue and may be an unique reagent for studying the function of various sialyl residue of cell surfaces.

The purified antibodies have the following advantages over lectins: 1) monovalent species (Fab) can be readily prepared.   2) antibodies or Fab fractions in the absence of complement are not cytotoxic in contrast to most lectins which are cytotoxic.   3) specificities of antibodies are better defined and narrower than that of lectins.

Reduction of cell growth rate and cell saturation density have been observed when NIL or NIL_{py} cells were cultured in the presence of antibodies against globoside(Laine and Hakomori, unpublished observation).

It is expected that results of surface labeling as described could be further assessed by "modification" of cell surfaces as described above, and these approaches will hopefully correlate biochemical events of phenotypic expression exerted on cell surfaces with the regulatory changes of genotypes during carcinogenesis and other physiological and pathological processes.

Fig. 7. *Synthesis of a globoside-sepharose complex.*

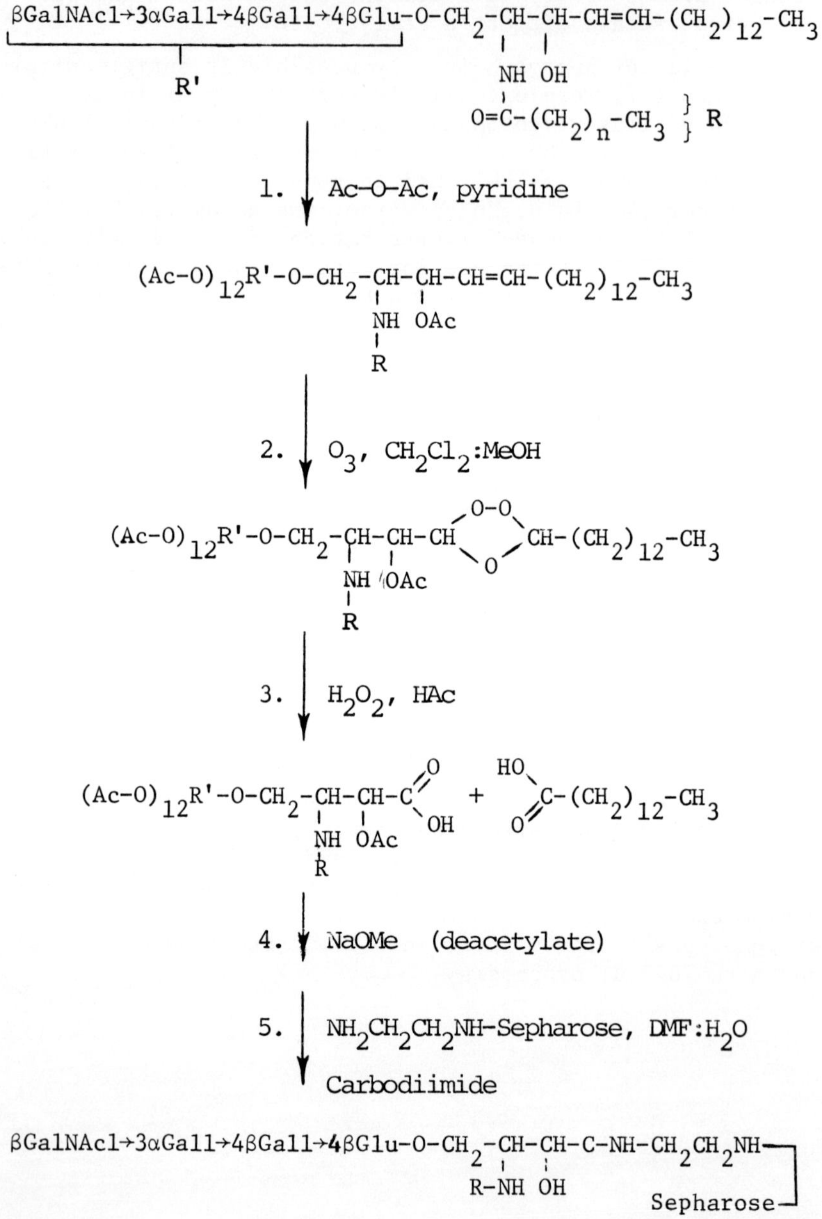

$$\underbrace{\beta GalNAc1 \rightarrow 3\alpha Gal1 \rightarrow 4\beta Gal1 \rightarrow 4\beta Glu}_{R'} - O-CH_2-\underset{\underset{O=\overset{|}{C}-(CH_2)_n-CH_3 \ \}}{\underset{NH}{|}}{CH}-\underset{\underset{OH}{|}}{CH}-CH=CH-(CH_2)_{12}-CH_3 \Bigr\} R$$

1. $\downarrow$ Ac-O-Ac, pyridine

$$(Ac-O)_{12}R'-O-CH_2-\underset{\underset{R}{\underset{|}{NH}}}{CH}-\underset{OAc}{\underset{|}{CH}}-CH=CH-(CH_2)_{12}-CH_3$$

2. $\downarrow$ O_3, CH_2Cl_2:MeOH

$$(Ac-O)_{12}R'-O-CH_2-\underset{\underset{R}{\underset{|}{NH}}}{CH}-\underset{OAc}{\underset{|}{CH}}-CH\overset{O-O}{\underset{O}{\diagdown}}CH-(CH_2)_{12}-CH_3$$

3. $\downarrow$ H_2O_2, HAc

$$(Ac-O)_{12}R'-O-CH_2-\underset{\underset{R}{\underset{|}{NH}}}{CH}-\underset{OAc}{\underset{|}{CH}}-C\overset{O}{\underset{OH}{\diagup}} + \overset{HO}{\underset{O}{\diagup}}C-(CH_2)_{12}-CH_3$$

4. $\downarrow$ NaOMe (deacetylate)

5. $\downarrow$ $NH_2CH_2CH_2NH$-Sepharose, DMF:H_2O

$\downarrow$ Carbodiimide

$$\beta GalNAc1 \rightarrow 3\alpha Gal1 \rightarrow 4\beta Gal1 \rightarrow 4\beta Glu-O-CH_2-\underset{\underset{R-NH}{\underset{|}{CH}}}{CH}-\underset{OH}{\underset{|}{CH}}-C-NH-CH_2CH_2NH-\Bigr] \text{Sepharose}$$

Fig. 8. *Synthesis of a hematoside-glass beads complex.*

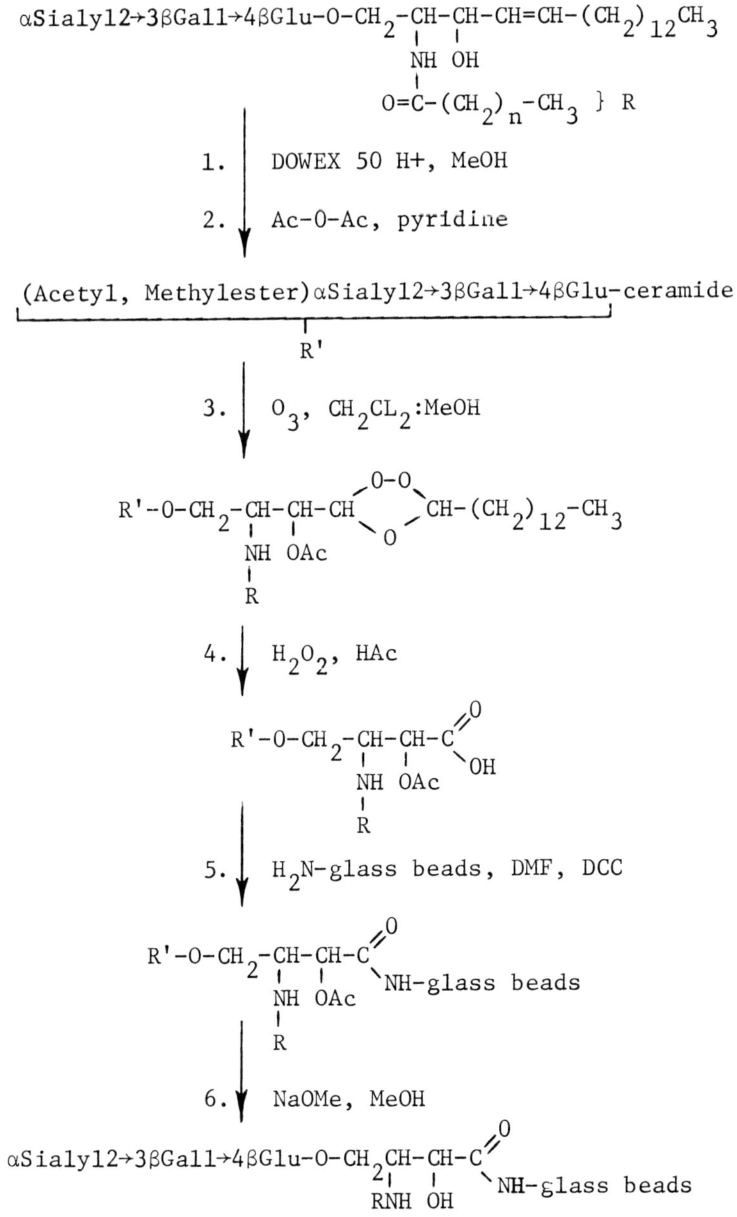

$$\alpha Sialyl2 \rightarrow 3\beta Gall \rightarrow 4\beta Glu-O-CH_2-CH-CH-CH=CH-(CH_2)_{12}CH_3$$

$$\begin{array}{c} | \quad | \\ NH \quad OH \\ | \\ O=C-(CH_2)_n-CH_3 \ \} \ R \end{array}$$

1. DOWEX 50 H+, MeOH

2. Ac-O-Ac, pyridine

(Acetyl, Methylester)$\alpha Sialyl2 \rightarrow 3\beta Gall \rightarrow 4\beta Glu$-ceramide

R'

3. O_3, CH_2CL_2:MeOH

$$R'-O-CH_2-CH-CH-CH \overset{O-O}{\underset{O}{\diagup}} CH-(CH_2)_{12}-CH_3$$

$$\begin{array}{c} | \quad | \\ NH \quad OAc \\ | \\ R \end{array}$$

4. H_2O_2, HAc

$$R'-O-CH_2-CH-CH-C \overset{\diagup O}{\underset{OH}{\diagdown}}$$

$$\begin{array}{c} | \quad | \\ NH \quad OAc \\ | \\ R \end{array}$$

5. H_2N-glass beads, DMF, DCC

$$R'-O-CH_2-CH-CH-C \overset{\diagup O}{\underset{NH-glass\ beads}{}}$$

$$\begin{array}{c} | \quad | \\ NH \quad OAc \\ | \\ R \end{array}$$

6. NaOMe, MeOH

$$\alpha Sialyl2 \rightarrow 3\beta Gall \rightarrow 4\beta Glu-O-CH_2CH-CH-C \overset{\diagup O}{\underset{NH-glass\ beads}{}}$$

$$\begin{array}{c} | \quad | \\ RNH \quad OH \end{array}$$

93

REFERENCES

(1)   D.F.H. Wallach, New Engl. J. Med., 280 (1969) 761.

(2)   S. Hakomori and W.T. Murakami, Proc. Nat. Acad. Sci. U.S.A., 59 (1968) 254.

(3)   S. Steiner, P.J. Brennan, and J.L. Melnick, Nature, 245 (1973) 19.

(4)   T. W. Keenan and D.J. Morré, Science, 182 (1973) 935.

(5)   S. Hakomori, Proc. Nat. Acad. Sci., 67 (1970) 1741.

(6)   L.A. Cumar, R.O. Brady, E.H. Kolodny, V.W. MacFarland, and P.T. Mora, Proc. Nat. Acad. Sci., 67 (1970) 757.

(7)   P.T. Mora, P.H. Fishman, R.H. Bassin, R.O. Brady, and V.W. MacFarland, Nature (New Biol.) 245 (1973) 226.

(8)   H. Den, A.M. Schultz, M. Basu, and S. Roseman, J. Biol. Chem., 246 (1971) 2721.

(9)   S. Kijimoto and S. Hakomori, Biochem. Biophys. Res. Commun., 44 (1971) 557.

(10) K. Stellner and S. Hakomori, Biochem. Biophys. Res. Commun., 55 (1973) 439.

(11) S. Hakomori, Colloq. Ges. Physiol. Chem., 22 (1971) 65.

(12) S. Hakomori, in: Advances in Cancer Research, Vol. 18, ed. S. Weinhouse (in press).

(13) T. Saito and S. Hakomori, J. Lipid Res., 12 (1971) 257.

(14) S. Hakomori, B. Siddiqui, Y.T.Li; S.C.Li, and C. G. Hellerquist, J. Biol. Chem., 246 (1971) 2271.

(15)   R.A. Laine C.C., Sweeley, Y.T.Li., A. Kisic,
         M.M. Rapport, J. Lipid Res., 13 (1972) 519.

(15a)   B. Siddiqui, J. Kawanami, Y.T. Li and S. Hakomori,
         J. Lipid Res. 13, (1972) 657.

(16)   K. Stellner, K. Watanabe, S. Hakomori, Biochemistry
         12 (1973) 656.

(17)   S. Hakomori, K. Stellner, K. Watanabe, Biochem.
         Biophys. Res. Comm., 49 (1972) 1061.

(18)   S. Basu, B. Kaufman, S. Roseman, J. Biol. Chem.,
         243 (1968) 5802.

(19)   J. Hildebrand, G. Hauser, J. Biol. Chem., 244 (1969)
         5170.

(20)   M. Goto and H. Sato, Gann, 63 (1972) 371.

(21)   J.K. Sheppard, Proc. Nat. Acad. Sci. 68 (1971) 1316.

(22)   H. Kalckar, D. Ullrey, S. Kijimoto, and S. Hakomori,
         Proc. Nat. Acad. Sci., 70 (1973) 839.

(23)   C.G. Gahmberg and S. Hakomori, J. Biol. Chem., 248
         (1973) 4311.

(24)   C.G. Gahmberg and S. Hakomori, Proc. Nat. Acad. Sci.,
         70 (1973) 3329.

(25)   R.H. Rice and G.E. Means, J. Biol. Chem., 246 (1971)
         831.

(26)   J. Folch, S. Arsove, and I. Heath, J. Biol. Chem.,
         191 (1951) 819.

(27)   C.C. Sweeley and B. Walker, Anal. Chem., 36 (1964)
         1461.

(28)   S. Hakomori, J. Koscielak, K.J. Block and R.W.
         Jeanloz, J. Immunl., 98 (1967) 31.

(29)   S. Hammarström and G. Bjursell, FEBS letters, 32
       (1973) 69.

(30)   C. Degani   and P.D. Boyer, J. Biol. Chem., 248,
       (1973) 8222.

(31)   S.P. Robins and A. J. Bailey, Biochem. Biophys.
       Res. Comm., 48 (1972) 1061.

(32)   L. Warren, D. Critchley, and I. MacPherson, Nature,
       235 (1972) 275.

(33)   L. Warren, J.B. Fuhrer, and C.A. Buck, Proc. Nat.
       Acad. Sci. U.S.A., 69 (1972) 1838.

(34)   C.G. Gahmberg, D. Kiehn, and S. Hakomori, Nature,
       in press (1974).

(35)   A.W. Hsie and T.T. Puck, Proc. Nat. Acad. Sci.,
       68 (1971) 358.

(36)   G. Johnson, R. Friedman, and I. Pastan, Proc. Nat.
       Acad. Sci., 68 (1971) 425.

(37)   G.L. Nielson and M. Lacorbiere, Proc. Nat. Acad.
       in U.S.A., 70 (1973) 1672.

(38)   B. Siddiqui and S. Hakomori, Cancer Res., 30 (1970)
       2930.

(39)   P. Gheema, G. Yogeeswaran, M.P. Morris, and R.K.
       Murray, FEBS Lett., 11 (1970) 181.

(40)   G. Yogeeswaran, R. Sheinin, J. Wherrett, and R.K.
       Murray, J. Biol. Chem., 247 (1972) 5146.

(41)   H. Diringer, G. Ströbel, and M.A. Koch, Hoppe-
       Seyler's Z. Physiol. Chem., 353 (1972) 1769.

(42)   H. Sakiyama and P.W. Robbins, Arch. Biochem.
       Biophys., 154 (1973) 407.

(43)   W.P. Wan Beek, L.A. Smets, and P. Emmelot, Cancer
       Res., 33 (1973) 2913.

(44) A. Vaheri, E. Ruoslahti, and S. Nordling, Nature New Biol. 238 (1972) 211.

(45) D. Marcus and L. Cass, Science 164 (1969) 553.

(46) R.A. Laine and S.Hakomori, Biochem. Biophys. Res. Commun. 54 (1973) 1039

(47) S. Hakomori, Methods of Enzymology, Volume 28, ed. by V. Ginsburg, Academic Press, (1973) 232.

(48) R.A. Laine and S. Hakomori, Fed. Proc. 32 (1973) 483, Abst. #1468.

(49) R.A. Laine, G. Yogeeswaran and S. Hakomori, J. Biol. Chem. (Submitted) 1974.

We wish to acknowledge National Institute of Health Grants CA 10909 and CA 12710 and American Cancer Society Grant BC-9D. Carl Gahmberg was supported by International Fogarty Center Fellowship 1 F05 TWO 1885-02.

DISCUSSION

G. Koch, Roche Institute of Molecular Biology: I have two questions. The gel pattern of glycoproteins obtained after incubation of transformed cells in the presence of cyclic AMP shows a new peak. In your recent paper in PNAS you referred to that peak and also to the fact that after incubation of transformed cells in the presence of cyclic AMP your gel pattern is different from the one found in normal cells. Does cyclic AMP induce the synthesis and accumulation of a specific glycoprotein in the cell membrane of transformed and of normal cells?

S. Hakomori, University of Washington: Well, at the moment, these surface labelled patterns are only preliminary results and we have to compare these label patterns under exactly the, same conditions. I'm not completely sure whether they're "induced patterns" or"normal patterns" or one of the phases of the surface during the cell growth, it's a kind of new pattern created by galactose and cyclic AMP.

G. Koch: My second question. We have studied the effect of polycations on protein synthesis in HeLa cells. Low concentrations of DEAE-dextran stimulate protein synthesis as measured by incorporation of labeled amino acids into proteins but high concentrations inhibit protein synthesis. Since you can revert the growth characteristics and glycoprotein patterns of transformed cells to resemble those of normal cells by incubation with the polyanion dextran sulfate, I ask you if anyone has done an experiment to see whether the growth characteristics and glycoprotein pattern of normal cells incubated in the presence of polycations would be altered and resemble then those of normal cells?

S. Hakomori: I didn't do that experiment.

S. Steiner, Baylor College of Medicine: I was wondering, Dr. Hakomori, if the galacto-protein that you see on the surface is present in any of the sub-cellular fractions, that is, mitochondria, nuclear membrane or endoplasmic reticulum?

S. Hakomori: I can't answer this question at the moment.

I. Macpherson, Imperial Cancer Research Fund Laboratories: We have fractionated iodinated cell membranes by nitrogen cavitation followed by separation in 10-60% sucrose gradients in a zonal centrifuge. The iodinated proteins are predominantly in plasma membrane vesicles (i.e., the fraction with the highest Na^+/K^+ ATPase activity). The soluble proteins have virtually no iodine label.

R. M. Roberts, University of Florida: When you were comparing the transformed cells with their counterparts treated with either galactose or cyclic AMP, weren't you in fact contrasting growing cells with cells that were not proliferating and possibly held predominantly in G_1? Therefore, aren't your comparisons invalid?

S. Hakomori: The effect of galactose is only limited to NILpy cells, so the possibility you mentioned can be excluded.

R. M. Roberts: Are the cells dividing?

S. Hakomori: No.

M. Horowitz, New York Medical College: Do you find any sloughing off or loss of glycolipids into the medium during the actively proliferative stages and secondly are there any effective lytic lipids such as lysolecithin present and do they induce changes in glycolipids? Have you observed anything like this?

S. Hakomori: No we haven't done that experiment.

M. Horowitz: How about the first one so far? Any loss into the medium of glycolipids during active proliferation?

S. *Hakomori*: No, I didn't do that experiment.

M. *Horowitz*: Thank you.

M. J. *Weber, University of Illinois*: You demonstrated some cell-cycle dependence of the exposure of cell-surface components, since you felt that these might be involved in the control of transport, I thought I'd make an additional comment. A student of mine, Arthur Hale, has examined hexose transport as a function of the cell cycle in chick cells. He finds no changes in hexose transport through the cell cycle, except for a small drop during the mitosis. Using cells infected with TS mutant of Rous sarcoma virus, he could also show that the induction of the transformed state was not cell cycle dependent. In these experiments he used hexose transport as a marker for the transformed state, and demonstrated that you could switch on hexose transport by a temperature shift at any stage in the cell cycle. This suggests that the structural changes which you show to be cell cycle dependent are not associated with at least this particular functional change.

S. *Hakomori*: Thank you very much. I don't think this is not simply cell cycle dependent, but as I said it's also contact dependent.

S. *Roseman, Johns Hopkins University*: Phil Robbins isn't here, or I would have asked him, but I thought his laboratory reported at the Federation meetings that there is no correlation between the normal state, transformed and tumorigenicity and the complexity of the lipids and the glycolipids. Is that wrong?

S. *Hakomori*: I'm sorry, my ear is bad.

S. *Roseman*: Perhaps Dr. MacPherson will answer the question.

I. *MacPherson*: The correlation still exists although Robbins has shown there are exceptions. It is not an absolute correlation.

S. Roseman: Well, if you start getting exceptions then you have to start worrying about the general rule, don't you.

I. MacPherson: Possibly, but there may be a number of points en route to a particular end result at which a defect can occur.

S. Hakomori: You're talking about the effect of cyclic AMP?

S. Roseman: No, I'm not...no. I'm talking about transformation, normal cell and tumorigenicity and lipids.

I. MacPherson: Glycolipid changes may be part of a train of events which finally precipitates DNA synthesis and cell division. The fact that this change is missing in some cell variants doesn't mean it is irrelevant in all cases. These variants could skip the glycolipid step and have their aberration somewhere else.

S. Roseman: But the key point, you see, as I understood it, in the early work was that here was a chemical change that always accompanied transformation, that was in fact characteristic of transformation. While there must be many ways to go to transformation, many branches to get to the final step, the final characteristic product should be the same.

I. MacPherson: I do not think one should lose interest because the correlation is not absolute. The commonest train of events which shows up as a correlation may involve a glycolipid change.

H. Eagle, Albert Einstein College of Medicine: I recently heard a seminar by Bob Pollack of the Cold Spring Harbor Laboratory, who has made this complicated question yet more complicated. With some ingenious selective procedures, he has succeeded in dissociating the decreased serum requirement of transformed cells, their ability to grow in agar, and the increased population density achieved in culture. At least with respect to these 3 properties there are clear dissociations, in that one may isolate transformants with one property, but not the other two.

He has not yet gotten to the key question as to which if any of these properties is rigorously associated with tumorigenecity.

I. MacPherson: I am beginning to repeat myself. All I am trying to say is that if a correlation breaks down when some exceptions are recognized, we should not assume that the correlated phenomena are unrelated.

S. Roseman: I think you're coming through. It means the take-home lesson is to stop working with tissue culture cells and stick with bacteria.

I. MacPherson: Well, if it turns you on, but I think you would be giving up a good opportunity to find out something about growth regulation in animal cells.

S. Roseman: I'm not so sure of that.

I. MacPherson: Can you offer a substitute? I know you are kidding but some people may think you're not.

C. G. Gahmberg, University of Washington: I would like to answer to Dr. Roseman's question. When you look at chemical levels of glycolipids this may be a very insensitive technique because we know that they are not only on the plasma membranes, where they are enriched but also in smaller quantities on other membranes. I think that by looking, for example, on surface exposed glycolipids and in correlating them with transformation of cells could be a more sensitive technique and this pattern seems to follow fairly well the behavior of the cells.

S. Hakomori: May I say something about tumorigenicity and glycolipid problem. This involves certainly some immunological process which can be related to degree of exposure, mobility of glycolipids in membrane and so on. If we could invent some sensitive methods to pick up the surface exposed group as natural lymphocytes do, this could lead to find clear correlation between tumorigenicity, surface structures, and glycolipids.

INTERCELLULAR COMMUNICATION THROUGH MEMBRANE JUNCTIONS AND CANCER ETIOLOGY

WERNER R. LOEWENSTEIN

Department of Physiology and Biophysics
University of Miami School of Medicine
Miami, Fla. 520875

Abstract: Normal cells in tissues or in culture make junctions that permit the passage of molecules directly from one cell interior to another. Certain cancer cells fail to make such permeable junctions. This defect is corrected when these cells are fused with normal ones; the resulting hybrid cells make permeable junctions while they contain the chromosome complement of both parent cells. The junctional correction in the hybrid cells is parallelled by correction of the *in vitro* growth control defect and, in at least one hybrid system, by a correction of tumorigenicity. Some of the hybrid cells lose part of the normal parental chromosome complement upon continued cultivation. Analysis of the segregants suggests that the junctional defect and the *in vitro* growth control defect are genetically related. (Genetic analysis of tumorigenicity is not yet complete.) A possible etiological role of the junctional defects in cancer is discussed and some simple models for production of uncontrolled growth by junctional defect are presented.

THE COMMUNICATING JUNCTIONAL PASSAGEWAYS

The cells of many tissues are interconnected at specialized junctions of their surface membranes, through which molecules can flow from one cell interior to another (1-3). Often all or most of the cells of an organ are so interconnected. This kind of intercellular communication (*junctional communication*) seems well suited for disseminating growth controlling molecules through an organ or a tissue.

Reduced to its essential elements, a communicating cell junction consists, besides ordinary (nonjunctional) cell membrane, of permeable *junctional membrane* that allows the passage of cellular molecules, and of *junctional seal* that insulates the interior of the connected cell system from the exterior (Fig. 1). The ensemble constitutes an effective cell-to-cell *passageway unit* through which molecules of a wide range of sizes can flow with little loss to the exterior; probably many parallel passageway units make up a junction (1).

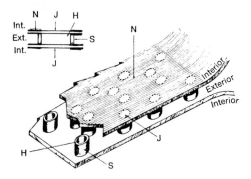

Fig. 1. Cell-to-cell passageways. *Top.* Diagram of a passageway unit, as defined by conductance measurements and by fluorescent tracer diffusion: *J,* Permeable *junctional membrane (J)* containing the "channels" for membrane diffusion; *N,* portions of relatively impermeable nonjunctional membrane; *S, junctional seal,* of unknown nature, circumscribing the intercellular aqueous "channel" *(H)* (From Loewenstein, 1966, ref. 1) *Bottom.* Schematic representation of a possible spatial relationship in a cell junction with extracellular space open to the exterior. Such a configuration allows two independent flows through the region of intercellular junction: one from cell-to-cell through the insulated passageway units and, perpendicular to this, another entirely extracellular (not dealt with in this paper). The tubular passageway configuration represented is one of several possibilities consistent with the studies of conductance and tracer diffusion.

These are the elements of a junction as they are defined by electrical measurement and by studies with intercellular fluorescent and colorant tracers. The structure of the elements is not known. A body of circumstantial (4-9) and genetic evidence (10) indicates that the "gap junction" (11), a junctional structure distinguishable in the electronmicroscope by an organized array of membrane particles (12-16), is a site of junctional communication in vertebrate cells (Fig. 2). It is possible that the membrane particles, which appear in register on the two adjoining membranes (12,14,17), contain the passageway units.

The most suggestive feature of a communicating junction concerning cellular growth control is that it permits the passage of molecules of the order of 500 MW and, in at least some instances, even larger ones. We were fortunate to find this out early (18, 19; see 2 for qualifications) and so, since then, had in sight the possibility that among the molecules passing through the junction may be some that control growth. This has all along been the working hypothesis of our research. I shall deal here with some of the results.

JUNCTIONAL COMMUNICATION AND GROWTH CONTROL

Potentialities. Before taking up the experiments, I shall look into some *a priori* arguments. It is not often necessary or even useful to give the reasoning behind a piece of work, because serendipity plays such a dominant role in biological research. Telling the outcome is usually enough. However, in the present instance, I think, a statement of *a priori* reasons may be useful.

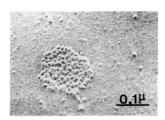

Fig. 2. Electronmicrograph of "gap junction" between two human skin fibroblasts. The cell membranes have been freeze-fractured at the junction, showing the typical junctional array of junctional particles. (Transections are shown in Fig. 4a, *right.*) (From Larsen, Azarnia & Loewenstein, unpublished.)

105

We start with the knowledge that in growth and differentiation of an organism, some form of cellular interaction at close range is at play. The past fifty years of experimental embryology have left this as a firm lesson. Here we have in junctional communication an obvious candidate for such close range interaction: a system in which molecules can diffuse directly from cell to cell with little loss. There are, of course, other close range forms of cellular interaction and, among these, communication by molecules diffusing through the extracellular fluid (humoral communication) or by molecules located on the cell surface membranes may play important roles in development. But junctional communication has unusual potential in developmental processes in which the number and position of cells is controlled. Because it is bounded by a sharp diffusion barrier --the barrier made of (nonjunctional) cell membrane and junctional seals -- the connected cell ensemble is a system of finite volume and hence has the potential of conveying information on cell number on the basis of simple properties of chemical concentration.[*] I shall illustrate this potential with a model.

A model for growth control. Consider a cell system connected by junctions, wherein each cell member (or member set) produces a burst of signal molecules and is sensitive to these molecules (Fig. 3). On the condition that the bursts occur asynchronously in the various cells, that the burst duration is small in relation to the burst intervals in each given cell, and that the molecules' diffusion time through the system is short in relation to the burst intervals in the various cells and to the time for diffusion out of the system, the steady state concentration of the signal molecules inside the cell system can provide information about the number of cells present in the system at that particular time: the mean concentration of the signal molecules simply is inversely proportional to the volume of the system, that is, approximately inversely proprotional to the number of cells in the system. Fed into an appropriate control loop, this information will regulate growth. For instance, if cell division proceeds only above a

---

[*] The sharp diffusion boundary confers also on the system the potential of providing information about the position of cells on the basis of time-dependent concentration parameters. For a model, see (2).

106

critical concentration of signal molecules, then division in a growing cell system will cease when the cells reach a number at which the signal molecules become diluted below the critical concentration. Such a system will curb cellular growth not only as the connected cell population increases by division (Fig. 3 A), but also when the population increases by establishment of junctional connection between formerly unconnected cells (Fig. 3 B) as, for example, between cells moving together in culture. In such systems, junctional obstruction or disconnection defeats growth control and, if the junctional defect is heritable, the result is a potentially cancerous system.

In terms of cancer, the junction in the foregoing model provides protection against excessive growth, by permitting dilution of the signal molecules in the interconnected cell system. This model was first proposed in 1968 (2). In an interesting alternative suggested by Socolar (20), the growth stimulating molecule is of extracellular origin and is taken up (via nonjunctional membrane) at rates that differ significantly from the norm in a few cells of the population. Here again a system connected by junctions permeable to the molecule can protect these cells, by signal dilution, against high signal concentration and, hence, against excessive growth; and as in the above model the result of junctional obstruction or disconnection is cancer. *The general condition for uncontrolled growth in both cases is that junctional transport of the signal molecule be sufficiently slowed in relation to the rates of signal production or of signal uptake.* This alternative is interesting in the light of Holley's (21) hypothesis that escape of transformed cells from growth control may be mediated by their excessive uptake of low-molecular-weight nutrients (see also 22, 23).

Variants of the model (with negative controls, time delays, etc.) or different models may be envisaged; a particularly interesting one has been proposed by Burton (24). I use the model of Fig. 3 here merely as an illustration of the power of a junctional system. The validity of this particular model is not essential to the argumentation in the following section.

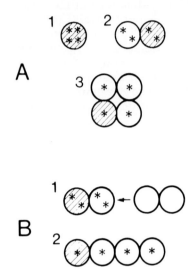

Fig. 3. A junctional model of growth control. Cells produce short, asynchronous bursts of signal molecules (∗) diffusing rapidly through the connected cell system. *A*, Growth by cell division. Diagrams of the cell system after two consecutive divisions (*2, 3*), at times when the molecules' concentration has reached steady state. The cell that produced the immediately preceding burst is shaded. The mean concentration provides each cell with the information of the size of the system. In the example represented, this information is used as a positive control signal: cell division proceeds so long as the concentration per cell is > 2 signal molecules. *B*, Growth by accretion. Two separate cell sets (*1*) join to form one system (*2*) (After Loewenstein 1968, ref. 2)

Junctional communication in developing organisms. The
second fact --a fact come to light over the past 7 years --
is the existence of widespread junctional communication in the
embryo. My colleague Ito (25) and, at Harvard, Potter,
Furshpan and Lennox (26) were the first to show this. Ito
showed that at the morula stage, most cells, probably all,
in the newt embryo are interconnected by junction; and the
Harvard group that, even at later stages of development, there
is extensive junctional communication between differentiating
groups of cells in the squid embryo. These results have been
confirmed for embryos of a broad variety of species (27-34).
We can thus be confident that junctional communication between different cell types and over long distances is a general
feature of embryonic organisms.

Defective Junctional Communication and Cancer

Etiology. All this, of course, is far from establishing an
involvement of junctional communication in growth control, or
even a correlation. It is merely the condition *sine qua non* for
such an involvement: the communication system is there when
controlled growth occurs.

How does one establish such a correlation? This would be
an easy task if we knew the growth controlling signal molecules. But the lack of knowledge of these signals is precisely
what hampers the whole field growth control and cancer. Thus
handicapped, the workers in the field are unable to take
direct approaches; and how hard it is, under such circumstances, to sort out significant etiological phenomena from epi-
phenomena, is all too obvious when one reads the literature
of cancer research.

My colleagues and I are in no way better off. We too had to
take an indirect approach, and only recently have we been
able to cut the risk that we may be chasing an epiphenomenon,
by the use of genetic analysis. Our general approach is to
search for defects in junctional communication among cancerous
tissues and to try to correlate the defects with cancerous growth
by genetic analysis. The rationale is as follows:

Control of growth, as does control of any system, requires
three elements: (*i*) the control signals, (*ii*) the receptor
(and effector) processes for these signals, and (*iii*) the means

of conveyance for these signals. Thus, in principle, uncontrolled growth, cancer, may arise by defects in (*i*) signal production, (*ii*) signal reception, and (*iii*) signal conveyance. Each of these defects constitutes a broad etiological category, each itself, in principle, a sufficient cause of cancer. Thus, *if the junction is indeed a path for growth-controlling molecules, then interruption or blockage of the path (uncoupling) by genetic defect should produce uncontrolled growth* (and this should be so regardless of the validity of the particular model of Fig. 3). This simple idea has guided our work into the cancer field.

Our focus is on category *iii.* The approach was first to search for junction-defective cells and, then, to attempt to relate the defect to the cancerous state. We have succeeded in the first, and are half-way in the second step.

Before describing the findings, I should like to say something about cancer cells that are *not* junction-defective. In the aforegoing view of cancer etiology, each of the three broad etiological categories constitutes *a* sufficient cause and, for the particular cancer form, *the* necessary cause of uncontrol. Thus, there is no reason to expect that cancer forms falling in category *i* and *ii* should have defective junction. This, to most readers, will be obvious. I stress it nonetheless, because some workers have shown confusion on this point. Their confusion stems probably from thinking of cancer as a single entity instead of what it is, a portmanteau for a diversity of forms of uncontrolled growth. In fact, we know now 7 kinds of cancer cells with no apparent qualitative junctional defect in respect to passage of inorganic ions and fluorescein (3,26,35-37); and there are undoubtedly more. This is not surprising or even interesting in terms of cancer etiology.

Junction-defective cancer cells. Our search for junction-defective cancer cells was encouraged by the results of physico-chemical studies on junctions, revealing that junctional communication is labile: it is susceptible to uncoupling by various chemical and physical means. For instance, inhibition of cell metabolism (38), prolonged exposure to Ca, Mg-free medium (39), substitution of Li for extracellular Na (39) or of propionate for extracellular Cl (40), anisotonicity (41,42), increase in the level of free cytoplasmic Ca^{++} (42-44), all produce uncoupling. We hoped, therefore, that

110

uncoupling due to genetic defect might occur frequently enough to give a reasonable chance of finding some kinds of noncoupling cancer cells.

We have found such cancer cells. We have isolated so far six strains of cells in culture which show no sign of junctional communication. Four of the strains were derived from rat hepatomas (35,45), one was produced by X-radiation of hamster embryo cells (35), and one is a malignant derivative of an L cell (10).[*] These cell strains contrast sharply by their junctional failure with normal cells. Normal cells in culture make junctions not only with cells of their own kind (3), but with cells of different organs and different tissues (51; see also 52). For instance, an epithelial cell from rabbit lens will couple to an epithelial cell from rat liver or to a fibroblast from hamster or man (51).

The cells of the six strains show no sign of making communicating junctions with cells of their own kind or with normal cells:(a) they fail to pass small inorganic ions (K^+, Cl^-, etc.) through junctions, as shown by electrical measurements with intracellular microelectrodes (10,35,45); (b) they fail to pass the larger exogenous molecule fluorescein (300 MW), as shown by studies in which the fluorescein anion is injected into the cells (10,45); and (c) they fail to pass endogenous nucleotide molecules or their derivatives, as shown by radioautographic studies on cells loaded with radioactive hypoxanthine (53). "Fail" must be understood in a qualified sense, since the experimental methods are, of course, limited in resolving power. But the resolving power of method a and , in some instances that of b, is high. Thus, if junctional communication is present at all in the strains, the rate of cell-to-cell diffusion of molecules must be several orders of magnitude smaller than in normal cells, and this may be functionally

---

[*] The present paper deals only with studies on cancer cells isolated in culture. Our earlier work on junctional communication in solid tumors is reviewed in (1) and (46). For studies on junctional structure in tumors, see (47-50).

equivalent to complete failure. * The six cell strains are also clearly defective in their growth patterns; *in vitro*, they do not show the density-dependent growth of normal cells and, in animals, they are highly tumorigenic.

Genetic correlation. Azarnia and I have now begun to analyze some of these cells genetically to find out whether the growth and junctional defects are related. We fuse cells from the noncoupling strain with normal cells and look to the ability of the hybrids to make communicative junctions and tumors. This approach was prompted by the findings of Weiss, Todaro and Green (54) and of Harris and Klein and colleagues (55,56) that density-dependent growth is resumed and tumorigenicity reduced in hybrids between various kinds of cancer and normal cells. This also turned out to be the case in our cell system. So the question was then whether the normalization of the growth properties is associated with normalization of junctional properties. The results in the three types of hybrid cell systems we have so far examined are simple: the correction of the growth defect is paralleled by a correction of the junctional defect.

---

* Our search was aimed at cells which, within the limits of the methods, are fully uncoupled. Among the various possible junctional defects, such a radical one seemed the easiest to determine. Here the electrical method can be used to its fullest advantage; an uncoupling determined by this method means that the junction is blocked to the passage of the small cellular inorganic ions (the carriers of the electrical current in the cells) and, therefore, probably to that of the larger cellular molecules. This presupposes that the inorganic ions and the larger permeant molecules normally take the same junctional route and that there is no preferential passage of uncharged molecules. At least the first is likely, since wherever the passages of inorganic ions and of fluorescein or other tracer molecules of comparable size were studied together, their block has been found to go hand in hand; this has been found for uncoupling produced by a variety of experimental procedures (19,39,43) as well as for uncoupling by certain genetic defects (10,35,57) where, passage has been found to be blocked not only for inorganic ions and fluorescein but also for some endogenous nucleotides or their derivatives (6,10).
It is, of course, entirely possible that there are also more

I shall report here briefly on the results obtained with two hybrid cell systems. In one system, the partners for fusion, the parent cells, were an epithelial *liver cell* and an epithelial *hepatoma cell* from rat. The initial contrast between the parent cells could not have been more striking: the liver cell is coupling, grows to densities of 10^4 cells/cm^2 in culture, and is not tumorigenic; the hepatoma cells is noncoupling, grows to densities $> 10^6$ cells/cm^2 in culture, and is highly tumorigenic (inocula of 10^2 cells produce fatal tumors). The hybrids --the primary products of cell fusion (heterokarya)--

subtle forms of uncoupling. For instance, the junctional passageways could be selectively blocked for a certain size or configuration of molecules and thus exclude the growth controlling molecules rather selectively (2); or the junctional passageway could be partly obstructed, reducing the rate of the junctional flow of the molecules below the minimum necessary for their adequate dissemination through the cell system and thus, as discussed above in terms of a particular model, bring about uncontrolled growth. Determination of uncoupling of the first kind is beyond the reach of the presently available methods. Determination of uncoupling of the second kind, if done with electrical method, would require precise measurement of electrical junctional and nonjunctional membrane resistances (in turn requiring selected cell systems of simple geometry). Moreover, to interpret meaningfully subtle quantitative differences of electric junctional resistance in terms of growth control in a cancer cell system, one may have to measure further parameters of the cell system that are related to molecular fluxes and dilution, in which context the differences in electrical resistance could be evaluated. Identification of such parameters will depend on the particular working model of growth control that one choses. For example, in the case of the model above, the topology of the cell population would have to be known. All this is technically difficult. Therefore, in the absence of knowledge on the identity and size of the growth-controlling molecules, it seemed to us more promising to put our bets on radical uncoupling in our search for junction-defective cancer cells.

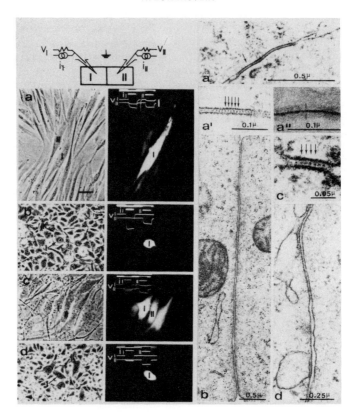

Fig. 4. Junctional communication and junctional structure in the human cell/mouse cell hybrid system. *a*, human parent cell; *b*, mouse parent cell; *c*, early hybrid between these cells, with nearly complete parent chromosome complement; *d*, revertant hybrid, after loss of about 30 of the 46 human chromosomes. *Left column*, properties of junctional communication: Current ($i = 1 \times 10^{-8}$ amp) is injected into cell I and, with a 100-msec delay, into cell II, and the resulting changes in membrane voltage (V) are measured simultaneously in the two cells with the aid of intracellular microelectrodes and displayed on an oscilloscope (*insets*). Simultaneously, fluorescein is injected into cell I and the fluorescence photographed 5 min thereafter. The relatively large V_2 in *a* and *c* show the cell-to-cell passage of small inorganic ions (the carriers of i), and the fluorescein spread shows the cell-to-cell passage of this 300-MW molecule. *Right column*,

as well as several generations of descendants of the heterokarya, took in all these respects after the normal liver cell
parent (57).

This is as far as we have gone with the liver cell/hepatoma
cell system. Here hybridization yielded rather stable chromosome combinations and, even after many months, there was
little sign of segregation.

We have taken the analysis further in another, less stable
cell system in which the parent cells are a coupling *human
cell* and a noncoupling *mouse cell* (10). The human cell is a
skin fibroblasts from a Lesh-Nyhan patient and the mouse cell,
a derivative (Cl-1D) of an L cell. This cell system is unusu-
ally suited for genetic analysis: the parent cells are genetically marked by enzyme defects permitting easy hybrid
selection, the karyotypes are readily distinguishable, and
the hybrids lose chromosomes at a rate appropriate for
segregant isolation. The system offers the additional advantage that the coupling human cell shows only one differentiated junctional structure in the electron microscope, namely
the "gap junction"; and that the noncoupling mouse cell
shows no distinguishable junctional structure at all (10). Thus
one can focus simultaneously on junctional permeability, gap-
junctional structure, and growth properties (Fig. 4).
However tests of tumorigenicity with such a heterologous
system are necessarily complex; because of this, our tumorigenicity tests are lagging behind.

The junction and growth properties of the parent cells,
in summary, are as follows:

The human cell is coupling, has gap junctions, and is

Fig. 4 (Continued)

electronmicrographic samples of transections of the junctions
between the corresponding cells. Gap junctions, with particles (arrows; *a, a'*) and typical "gap" after Lanthanum
infiltration (*a"*); and between two early hybrids (*c*). Typical
undifferentiated junction between two mouse parent cells (*b*)
and two revertant cells (*d*). (From Azarnia, Larsen &
Loewenstein 1974, ref. 10.)

density-dependent in its growth *in vitro*. The mouse cell is noncoupling, lacks gap junction (I shall call these two defects collectively *junction-defective trait*) and is not density-dependent*

The hybrids between these cells took in all these respects after the human parent, while they contained the nearly complete parent chromosome complement (Fig. 4c). Upon continued cultivation, the hybrid cells tended to lose chromosomes, preferentially the human ones. This is a common feature of this parent cell combination (54). As the hybrid cells lost the human chromosomes, clones appeared which had reverted to the junction-defective and growth-defective traits of the mouse parent (Fig. 4d). In all such revertant clones, the junction-defective trait went associated with the growth-defective one, although the junction defect and growth defect had segregated from a number of other traits which originally occurred together in the mouse parent cell (10).

These results suggest a genetic correlation between defective junctional communication and defective growth pattern *in vitro*: the results reveal that the human cell contributes a genetic factor to the hybrids, which corrects the junctional defect and the growth defect. This factor is probably linked to one or more human chromosomes, since loss of human chromosomes in the hybrids resulted in the reversion to both deficiencies. What remains now to be shown is whether the correlation extends also to the growth control deficiency *in vivo*, as we know it does in at least the unsegregated hybrids of the liver/hepatoma cell system (57). This we should know as soon as our tumorigenicity tests are completed.

---

* The mouse cell is, besides, tumorigenic and the human cell, nontumorigenic.

REFERENCES

(1)   W. R. Loewenstein. Ann. N.Y. Acad. Sci. 137 (1966) 441.

(2)   W. R. Loewenstein. Devel. Biol. 19 (Suppl.2) (1968) 151.

(3)   E. J. Furshpan & D. D. Potter. Curr. Top. Devel. Biol. 3 (1968) 95.

(4)   G. D. Pappas and M.V.L. Bennett. Ann. N.Y. Acad. Sci. 137 (1966) 495.

(5)   J. P. Revel, A. G. Yee and A. J. Hudspeth. Proc. Nat. Acad. Sci. 68 (1971) 2924.

(6)   N.B. Gilula, O.R. Reeves and A. Steinbach. Nature 235 (1972) 262.

(7)   P. Satir and N.B. Gilula. Ann. Rev. Entomol. 18 (1973) 143.

(8)   R.L. DeHaan and H.G. Sachs. Curr. Top. Devel. Biol. 8   (1973) 193.

(9)   N. McNutt and R. S. Weinstein. Prog. Biophys. Mol. Biol. 26 (1973) 45.

(10) R. Azarnia, W. Larsen and W.R. Loewenstein. Proc. Nat. Acad. Sci. 71 (1974) 880.

(11) J.P. Revel and M.J. Karnovsky. J. Cell Biol. 33 (1967) C7.

(12) J.P. Chalcroft and S. Bullivant. J. Cell Biol. 47 (1970) 49.

(13) D. A. Goodenough and J.P. Revel. J. Cell Biol. 45 (1970) 272.

(14) N.S. McNutt and R.S. Weinstein. J. Cell Biol. 47 (1970) 666.

(15) L.A. Staehelin. Proc. Nat. Acad. Sci. 69 (1972) 1318.

(16) C. Peracchia. J. Cell Biol. 57 (1973) 66.

(17) D. A. Goodenough. personal communication

(18) W.R. Loewenstein and Y. Kanno. J. Cell Biol. 22 (1964) 565.

(19) Y. Kanno and W.R. Loewenstein. Nature (1966) 212.

(20) S. J. Socolar. Exp. Eye Res. 15 (1973) 643.

(21) R. W. Holley. Proc. Nat. Acad. Sci. 69 (1972) 1840.

(22) A. B. Pardee. Nat. Cancer Inst. Monogr. 14 (1964) 7.

(23) C. L. Markert. Cancer Res. 28 (1968) 1908.

(24) A.C. Burton. Persp. Biol. Med. 14 (1971) 301.

(25) S. Ito and N. Hori. J.Gen. Physiol. 49 (1966) 1019.

(26) D.D. Potter, E.J. Furshpan and E.G. Lennox. Proc. Nat. Acad. Sci. 55 (1966) 328.

(27) J. Sheridan. J. Cell Biol. 37 (1968) 650.

(28) D.J. Woodward. J. Gen. Physiol. 52 (1968) 509.

(29) C. Slack and J.P. Palmer. Cell Res. 55 (1969) 416.

(30) M.V.L. Bennett and J.P. Trinkaus. J. Cell Biol. 44 (1970) 592.

(31) A.E. Warner. J. Physiol. 210 (1970) 150P.

(32) J.T. Tupper, J.W. Saunders and C. Edwards. J. Cell Biol. 46 (1970) 187.

(33) K. Takahashi, S. Miyazaki and Y. Kidokoro. Science 171 (1971) 415.

(34) J.T. Tupper and J.W. Saunders. Devel. Biol. 27 (1972) 546.

(35) C. Borek, S. Higashino and W.R. Loewenstein, J. Membrane Biol. 1 (1969) 274.

(36) J. Sheridan. J.Cell Biol. 45 (1970) 91.

(37) R.G. Johnson and J.D. Sheridan. Science 174 (1971) 717.

(38) A.L. Politoff, S.J. Socolar and W.R. Loewenstein. J. Gen. Physiol. 53 (1969) 498.

(39) B. Rose and W.R. Loewenstein. J. Membrane Biol. 5 (1971) 20.

(40) Y. Asada, G.O. Pappas and M.V.L. Bennett. Fed. Proc. 26 (1967) 330.

(41) L. Barr, W. Berger and D. Dewey. J. Gen. Physiol. 48 (1965) 797.

(42) W.R. Loewenstein, M. Nakas and S.J. Socolar. J. Gen. Physiol. 50 (1967) 1865.

(43) G.M. Oliveira-Castro and W.R. Loewenstein. J. Membrane Biol. 5 (1971) 51.

(44) B. Rose and W.R. Loewenstein. Science (1974) (in press).

(45) R. Azarnia and W.R. Loewenstein. J. Membrane Biol. 6 (1971) 368.

(46) W.R. Loewenstein. Arch. Intern. Med. 129 (1972) 299.

(47) E.L. Benedetti and P. Emmelot. J. Cell Sci. 2 (1967) 499.

(48) A. Martinez-Palomo, A. Brarslovsky, W. Bernard. Cancer Res. 29 (1969) 925.

(49) A. Martinez-Palomo. Lab. Invest. 22 (1970) 605.

(50)   R.S. Weinstein. This volume.

(51)   W. Michalke and W.R. Loewenstein. Nature 232 (1971)
       121.

(52)   R.G. Johnson, W.S. Herman and D.M. Preus.
       J. Ultrastructure Res. 43 (1973) 298.

(53)   R. Azarnia, W. Michalke and W.R. Loewenstein. J.
       Membrane Biol. 10 (1972) 247.

(54)   M.C. Weiss, J. Todaro and H. Green. J. Cell Physiol.
       71 (1968) 105.

(55)   G. Klein,A.F. Bregula,F. Wiener and H. Harris. J.
       Cell Sci. 8 (1971) 659.

(56)   H. Harris. Proc.R.Soc.Lond.B. 179 (1971) 1.

(57)   R. Azarnia and W.R. Loewenstein. Nature 241 (1973)
       455.

DISCUSSION

P. A. Srere, Veterans Administration Hospital: Do you know anything about the diffusion characteristics of the gap junction as opposed to the diffusion characteristics of the body of the cell. Are there differences in diffusion coefficients of your substance through the gap junction compared to its diffusion coefficient through the cell?

W. R. Loewenstein, University of Miami: I can't give you an answer in terms of diffusion constants. But I could try to do so in terms of conductance measurements, from which one could derive diffusion constants for the small inorganic ions, the carriers of the electrical current in our measurements. The estimates of junctional resistance in various cell systems range from 10^{-1} to 10^{1} Ωcm^2. This resistance is several orders of magnitude lower than that of nonjunctional membrane, but it is still greater than the resistance of a membrane made of cytoplasm. As to diffusion rates of larger molecules, we have no data available. It is hard to make accurate measurements of diffusion rates in small systems with irregular geometry. If a qualitative statement helps you at all, I could say that diffusion is fast for a molecule of 300MW, like fluorescein; fluorescein takes on the order of seconds to diffuse along a chain of cells containing 4-6 junctions.

P. A. Srere: Did I understand you to say that there was no electrical connection before you injected the dye, that you needed the dye to see the electrical response?

W. R. Loewenstein: Oh, not at all. The dye is simply a useful fluorescent probe of junctional permeability. As a matter of fact, junctional communication between nonexcitable cells was originally found by electrical measurement alone.

I. MacPherson, Imperial Cancer Research Fund Laboratories: From your studies with the human/mouse hybrid revertants, has it been possible to assign the coupling function to any particular group of human chromosomes?

W. R. Loewenstein: Not yet, unfortunately. We don't have enough segregants. In principle it should be possible to identify the chromosome or chromosomes that determine the coupling function. We hope to have enough segregants in a few more months to do this.

H. Brandt, University of Miami: On the last slide you correlated malignancy with cell population per cubic cm with conductance and showed the reversion after so many generations have elapsed, did you, or could you look at the rate that each of these two parameters were changing and see that the rates were the same?

W. R. Loewenstein: Sorry, I don't quite understand your question. But one thing I understood and that is wrong: my last slide did not deal with malignancy. Our malignancy tests on the mouse/human system are not yet completed. Our results in this system so far show only a correlation between the junctional defect and the in vitro growth defect of lack of density-dependent growth. It will take longer to find out whether there is such a simple correlation with malignancy. Tests of tumorigenicity with heterologous systems, involving negative results, are tedious and long.

S. Greer, University of Miami: You mentioned that lithium has an effect on these gap junctions. I wondered if anyone is looking into the possibility that this may explain the psycho-pharmalogical effect of lithium?

W. R. Loewenstein: Could you repeat that?

S. Greer: You mentioned that lithium affects the gap junction. It is known that lithium has a psycho-pharmalogical effect of unknown molecular basis.

W. R. Loewenstein: A psycho-?

S. Greer: Yes, anti-depressant actually anti-schizoid as well. It has been reported to have dramatic effects in psychiatric disorders.

W. R. Loewenstein: Oh, yes, I don't know. The only thing I could say is that in nerve cells, as shown by Baker, Hodgkin, Blaustein, and colleagues, substitution of lithium for extracellular sodium causes cytoplasmic free calcium to rise. One may reasonably expect therefore in an electrically coupled nerve cell, that synaptic electrical transmission be blocked as a result of the rise in calcium ions. The fact is that such substitution does cause uncoupling in epithelial cell junctions. Whether such uncoupling is at the root of the central-nervous-system phenomenon you are mentioning, is hard to say. There are many other possibilities, I am sure, in the case of such a complex phenomenon.

J. Roth, Biocenter: I was wondering if you see any effect of culture density on the formation of these junctions; for instance do you see these junctions in cultures of very low density?

W. R. Loewenstein: In very low density?

J. Roth: Perhaps 0.1 to 0.2 x 10^4 cells per cm squared.

W. R. Loewenstein: Say that again. What was the cell density?

J. Roth: The density? 0.1 to 0.2 x 10^4 cells per cm squared.

W. R. Loewenstein: One gets junction formation even if you have just a couple of cells. You just need them to get in contact.

J. Roth: But if they're very far apart, I was saying, if you see the cells at a very low density, do you see these junctions?

W. R. Loewenstein: You get junction formation even with only 2 cells in the whole dish, so long as they are in contact.

123

J. Roth: But how far apart, how close together do they have to be?

W. R. Loewenstein: Oh, they have to be in contact of course.

J. Roth: The phenomenon I was wondering about was if you see cells at a very low density there is a very marked inhibition of growth sometimes, similar to a lag phase that comes before logarithmic growth in normal cells; it wouldn't seem to agree with the idea that if you didn't have these junctions then you would have increased the amount of growth. It would seem to indicate that there are other factors aside from the conveyance of signals through junctions, that there must be something else, perhaps a necessity for growth signal commands before you have a shutoff mechanism; it must be more complicated, otherwise you would see very much more growth in cells that didn't have these junctions, expecially with low densities. But you do see this lag of growth and it doesn't seem....

W. R. Loewenstein: These cells, at low density, don't shut off growth?

J. Roth: The cells at very low density have a lag phase. They take approximately 24 to 36 hours before they start dividing after you've seeded them, whereas normally you don't have such a large lag, i.e., if you seed them at very low density. We've done this many times. We're particularly interested in this lag phase of growth because there are other things happening at that point, but one of the very consistent observations is that their growth is inhibited when you seed them at a very low density as opposed to seeding them at 1×10^4 where you see that the cells are soon close enough for cell junction. When they're not close enough for cell junction, then there is an inhibition of growth. My point there is that there must be some other factors involved.

W. R. Loewenstein: You are equating your "lag phase" to density inhibition of growth. Is this justified, or are there entirely different growth mechanisms involved? I have really nothing to say about such a "lag phase", except that you are wrong in supposing that at densities of

1×10^4 cells/cm^2, the cells are not close enough for making junctions. Junctions are often made by fine and long processes even at lower densities.

QUANTITATION OF OCCLUDENS, ADHERENS, AND NEXUS CELL JUNCTIONS IN HUMAN TUMORS

Ronald Weinstein, Gerald Zel and
Frederick B. Merk

Departments of Pathology and Urology
Tufts University School of Medicine

Abstract: Many solid tumors are characterized by decreases in intercellular adhesiveness and a loss of low resistance electrotonic coupling. Cell junctions bear part of the responsibility for these functions. The ultrastructure and frequency of various types of cell junctions (e.g., occludens, adherens, nexus, etc.) have been determined in two tumor systems, squamous cell tumors of the uterine cervix and transitional cell tumors of the urinary bladder. As described elsewhere (McNutt, Hershberg and Weinstein, J. Cell Biol. 51 [1971] 805), maculae adherentes and nexuses are present in large numbers (hundreds per cell) in normal squamous epithelium of the uterine cervix. In cervical carcinoma in situ, a preinvasive malignant state, maculae adherentes and nexuses are markedly reduced in frequency. Parallel reductions in junctional frequencies are observed in invasive squamous cell carcinoma of the cervix. In a tumor system described in this paper, junctional frequency is relatively unaltered in early stages of "malignant transformation." Normal transitional cell epithelium (urothelium) contains moderate numbers of maculae adherentes throughout the epithelium, and small numbers of nexuses. In carcinoma in situ and in low grade transitional cell carcinomas, the number of <u>maculae</u> <u>adherentes</u> junctions and <u>nexuses</u> is relatively unaltered. Thus, in the two tumor systems systematically examined to date, cell junction frequency behaves in a linked manner during tumorigenesis. Implications of this observation are discussed.

INTRODUCTION

Cells in normal epithelia are interadherent and may interact at short range to form metabolically cooperative tissues. Specialized sites (e.g., cell junctions) in the membranes of neighboring epithelial cells provide part of the structural basis for these tissue functions. The ultrastructure of cell junctions in mammalian tissues has been the subject of a recent comprehensive review (1). In brief, several Latin words are used to describe the configuration (shape and total area) of cell junctions (2). The term "zonula" is used where the junction extends as a belt around the entire cell (Fig. 1). "Fascia" is used when the junction is an extensive sheet-like area of attachment and "macula" is used when the junction is a simple spot or disk-shaped area. These terms describe configuration only and do not determine the general class into which junctions fall.

The major types of junctions that occur in many mammalian epithelia are occludens, nexus and adherens junctions (1,2). Some features of these junctions are illustrated in a schematic fashion in Figure 2.

All types of cell junctions contribute to intercellular adhesion. One type of junction, the occludens, provides a permeability barrier against by-pass diffusion (1,2) and another type of junction, the nexus (i.e., "gap" junction) is traversed by small conduits that provide passageways for ions and small molecules, enabling them to travel from cell to cell without entering the extracellular compartment (3-6).

CELL JUNCTION NOMENCLATURE

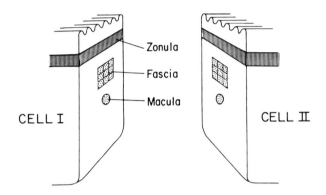

Fig. 1. Cell junction nomenclature. The terms "zonula", "fascia" and "macula," are used to describe the geometry of a junction in the plane of the cell membrane.

TYPES OF CELL JUNCTIONS

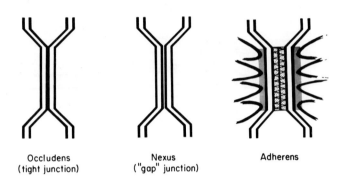

| Occludens | Nexus | Adherens |
| (tight junction) | ("gap" junction) | |

Fig. 2. Highly schematic representation of several types of cell junctions, as they appear in thin sections. The occludens (left) is characterized by focal union of the outer leaflets of the surface membranes of neighboring cells. The nexus (center) has a narrow gap separating the trilaminar "unit membranes" of each cell. At the adherens junction (right), the cell membranes are separated by a 15-35 nm space that contains electron-dense material. Dense plaques are subjacent to the membranes. In some tissues, tonofilaments may insert into the dense plaques.

Cell-to-cell adhesion and short range intercellular communication probably serve important roles in the control of normal differentiation and growth (7,8). Many malignancies show decreases in cellular adhesiveness (9,10) and loss of cell-to-cell electrotonic coupling (11,12). The abnormal intercellular adhesion and communication which is often exhibited by tumors may correlate well with structural abnormalities in their junctions (13-16).

The precise relationships of membrane surface components such as cell junctions to the
biological behavior of tumors (e.g., growth, invasion, and metastasis) are unknown. As part of
an effort to assess the roles played by junctions
in benign and malignant tumors, we have examined
the ultrastructure and frequency of junctions in
several tissues and are currently attempting to
correlate these parameters with the biological
behavior of the neoplastic epithelium. Efforts
have been focused on two organs, the human uterine cervix, as described elsewhere (14,15), and
the human urinary bladder, as described in this
communication. The use of solid tumors in
structure-function studies of malignant behavior
offers several advantages over the use of tissue
culture systems. Epithelia in many human organs
can exist in a number of pathological states that
may represent intermediate stages in malignant
evolution (17). Reasonable predictions concerning future biological behavior can be based on
available data regarding the natural history of
human tumors. Another advantage offered by some
human neoplasms is that certain aspects of tumorigenesis can be followed in individual patients.
For example, transitional cell carcinomas tend to
recur, usually in different locations within the
bladder, and become increasingly aggressive with
time. Patients with a history of bladder tumor
submit to periodic cystoscopy. This facilitates
the observation of alterations in the structure
and biological behavior of bladder epithelium
over a period of time (18).

EXPERIMENTAL

Collection of Tumors

Tumors of the human urinary bladder were obtained at cystectomy or by transurethral endo-
scopic resection. Fifteen specimens representing
various malignant states have been examined by
electron microscopy. These include cases of benign papilloma, carcinoma in situ, as defined by

Utz, et al. (19), and examples of papillary transitional cell carcinoma. Biopsies of bladder epithelium removed at surgery for non-malignant disease served as controls.

Electron Microscopy

Surgical specimens were divided. A portion was processed for routine diagnostic histopathology and the remainder was used for electron microscopy. Specimens were fixed in cold 2% glutaraldehyde in 0.1 M sodium cacodylate buffer, pH 7.4. Specimens for thin section electron microscopy were post-fixed in a 1% osmic acid in cacodylate buffer. Selected tissue blocks were stained en bloc with 1% uranyl acetate in Veronal buffer, pH 5.0, for 1 hour (20). Tissue blocks were dehydrated by passage through a graded series of water-ethanol solutions, infiltrated with Epon 812, and polymerized in a 60°C oven. Thin sections were cut on diamond knives, stained consecutively with uranyl acetate and lead citrate, and photographed in a Philips EM 300 electron microscope.

The freeze-cleave technique was performed as described by Moor (21). For cryoprotection, tissue blocks were soaked in 20% glycerol or 1 M Sucrose, buffered to pH 7.4 and rapidly cooled in Freon 22 to -150°C. Replicas were prepared in a Balzers BAF 301 freeze-etch device. They were separated from tissues with Clorox , washed with distilled water, picked up on 300 mesh coated grids and examined in the electron microscope.

Histopathological Grading and Staging of Tumors

A part of each biopsy was processed for routine light microscopic histopathological evaluation. Tumors were classified according to the grading system of the American Registry of Bladder Tumors. This system is composed of three numerical grades plus benign papilloma. Grade 1 transitional cell carcinoma is defined as a tumor

having a thickened epithelium displaying a minor
degree of anaplasia. Grade 2 carcinoma shows a
more anaplastic epithelium and a loss of cell
polarity with respect to the surface. In Grade 3
carcinoma, the transitional epithelium may not be
readily identified as such since the cells are
anaplastic and often bizarre (22,23). Tumors
were staged according to extent of bladder wall
infiltration and metastasis, according to the
criteria of Jewett and Strong (23).

Summary of Data on Junctions in Neoplastic Cervical Epithelium

Junctional frequencies have been quantitated
in a spectrum of neoplastic lesions arising in
the epithelium of the human uterine cervix (14,
15). In normal cervical epithelium, cell junctions are abundant, with several hundred nexuses
and maculae adherentes occuring on each cell in
the intermediate cell layer. Both types of junctions are markedly reduced in number in preinvasive malignant epithelia (e.g., carcinoma in
situ) and in invasive squamous cell carcinomas.
Relatively mild reductions in junction frequency
were noted in several non-malignant pathological
states. Since carcinoma in situ can be present
for long time intervals before an invasive lesion
arises from the cervical epithelium (25), these
results indicate that junctional deficiencies,
per se, do not cause stromal invasion by the
tumor (15).

Ultrastructure of Normal Human Bladder Epithelium (Urothelium)

Human urothelium is usually four to five
cells thick. The basal and intermediate cell
layers contain small cells that have a simple cytoarchitecture. The luminal surface of the bladder is lined by large polyploid cells that contain small numbers of distinctive fusiform vacuoles that are rimmed by an asymmetric unit membrane (26). Luminal cells are joined together

133

by zonulae occludentes junctions (27,28) and by
small, well formed maculae adherentes. Cells in
the basal and intermediate layers are joined together by small incomplete maculae adherentes
(29,30). Nexuses are encountered very infre-
quently in normal urothelium. The apparent
sparseness of the nexus population may correlate
well with the observation that small numbers of
bladder urothelial cells are electrotonically
coupled (31).

Cell Junctions in Neoplastic States of Bladder Urothelium

Changes in junctional frequency accompanying
tumorigenesis of bladder urothelium differ from
the changes in human cervical epithelium that
were described previously (15). In bladder urothelium there is an increase in the number of
maculae adherentes in low grade papillary transitional cell carcinomas (this study, 32,33) and in
carcinomas in situ. This increase is in contrast
to a decrease in frequency of maculae adherentes
found in analogous lesions of cervical epithelium. Nexus junctions are also present in tumors
of the bladder (Fig. 3). Because of the low frequency of nexuses in normal bladder, it is difficult to determine their relative frequency in a
statistically significant manner, but it is our
impression that nexuses are as frequent in carcinoma in situ and in low grade invasive lesions as
they are in normal bladder urothelium. The frequency of maculae adherentes and nexuses in
higher grade malignancies of the bladder has not
been determined in this study, but Fulker et al.
(32) report a decrease in maculae adherentes in
such tumors. No mention is made of nexus junctions in low or high grade malignancies in their
report.

Zonulae occludentes junctions are not present in cervical squamous epithelium. They are
present in normal bladder epithelium and in low

grade tumors (Fig. 4). Zonulae occludentes
junctions are incomplete in carcinoma in situ and
in higher grade malignancies of the bladder (32).

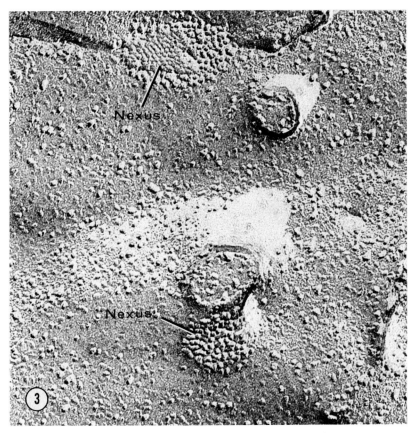

Fig. 3. Freeze-cleave electron microscopy
of two nexus junctions at the surface of a tumor cell in a human Grade 2 papillary transitional cell carcinoma. In freeze-cleave preparations, nexuses are characterized by distinctive arrays of 5-7 nm in diameter intramembranous subunits. X 117,000.

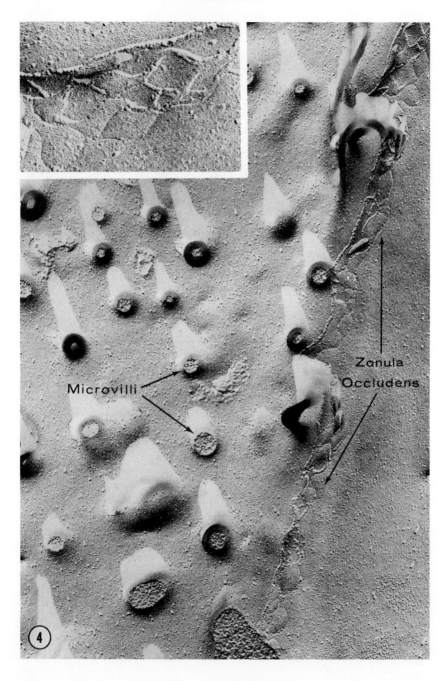

Fig. 4. Zonula occludens of a Grade 1 papillary transitional cell carcinoma in the human
urinary bladder. This type of junction joins
the lateral surfaces of two superficial cells
just below the luminal surface. Luminal micro-
villi, which cast long shadows in freeze-cleave
preparations, are seen at the left of the junction. The lateral surface of the cell is relatively flat (right). X 57,600. Insert: Detail
of Figure 4. Occludens junction is characterized by anastomosing ridges and grooves.
X. 126,000.

Hemidesmosomes: Possible Evidence of Qualitative
Defects in Tumor Junctions.

The morphogenesis of symmetrical desmosomes
(maculae adherentes), found within an epithelium,
involves: 1- the accumulation of electron dense
fibrils between the surfaces of neighboring cells;
2- condensation of finely filamentous material
into dense plaques beneath the surface membranes
of the cell pair forming the desmosome; and 3-
development of an intracellular system of fibrils
(e.g., tonofilaments) some of which may loop
through the dense plaques (34,35) (Fig. 5).   A
similar sequence of events occurs at the dermal-
epithelial front in skin and results in the formation of an asymmetrical junction, the hemidesmosome (35,36), which resembles the desmosome
but is at a cell surface where it abuts into the
stroma.   We are unaware of reports of hemidesmosomes within normal epithelia.

DEVELOPMENT OF DESMOSOMES

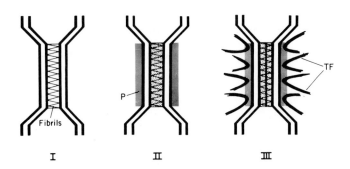

Fig. 5.   Morphogenesis of the desmosomes
(maculae adherentes).   Dense plaques (P) and
tonofilaments (TF) appear during desmosome
maturation (see text).

An unexpected finding in benign papilloma,
carcinoma in situ and low grade transitional cell
carcinomas of the bladder is the presence of hemidesmosomes within the epithelium (Figs. 6,7).
These asymmetric junctions have a fully developed
dense plaque subjacent to the cell surface membrane of one cell but not that of its neighbor.
Tonofilaments may loop through the single dense
plaque. Within the extracellular space is a condensation of finely fibrillar electron dense material. The mechanism of formation of these unusual structures is not known for certain. They
may arise by any one of several mechanisms: 1-in
vivo shearing of structurally defective symmetrical desmosomes; 2- incomplete desmosome formation
which could result from the failure of one cell
to assemble its contribution to the junction or;
3- as part of a cell dissociation-reassociation
cycle (34). The first two possibilities imply
that the junctions are structurally defective although the precise nature of the defect is inap-
parent by thin section electron microscopy. It
is also possible that the hemidesmosomes represent an artifact that is introduced by the electron microscopy preparative techniques. However,
we have been unable to demonstrate similar structures in normal urothelium or in high grade tumors.

Linked Behavior of Junctional Frequencies in Tumors

In the tumor systems investigated thus far,
the frequencies of several types of cell junctions
may change in a linked or coordinate manner with
tumorigenesis. In cervical epithelium, maculae
adherentes and nexuses are profoundly decreased
in carcinoma in situ and in invasive carcinoma
regardless of the grade of malignancy. On the
other hand, in bladder epithelium the frequency
of the same types of junctions in carcinoma in
situ and in low grade transitional cell carcinoma
is unchanged when compared with the frequency
found in normal bladder epithelium. Thus, frequencies of several types of junctions appear to
be influenced in a linked manner by tumorigenesis

and the direction of change appears to be tissue specific.

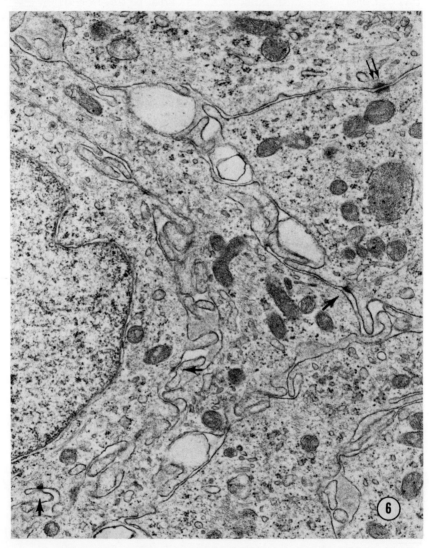

Fig. 6. Benign papilloma in human urinary bladder. A desmosome (double arrow) and three hemidesmosomes (single arrows) are present in this field. X 24,300.

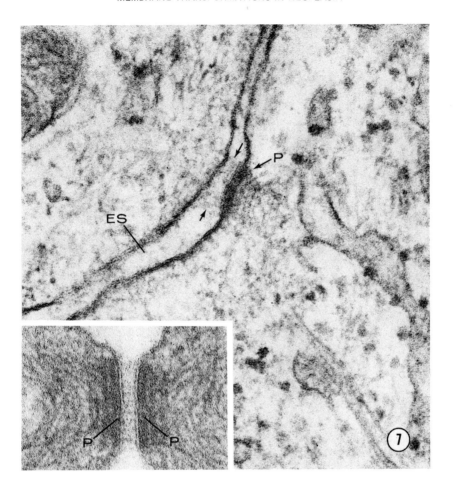

Fig. 7. Hemidesmosome in a benign papilloma (detail of Fig. 6). Areas of two neighboring cells are separated by the extracellular compartment (ES), which contains finely fibrillar material (arrows). An electron dense plaque (P) is subjacent to the surface membrane of one cell. X 122,400. Insert: Desmosome (macula adherens) in a human Grade 2 papillary transitional cell carcinoma. At the membranes of each of the neighboring cells dense plaques are present which are laced with tonofilaments. X 122,400.

Cell junction assembly mechanisms are not completely understood but available evidence is consistent with an hypothesis that they are assembled within the nonjunctional plasma membrane. For example, all types of junctions share certain ultrastructural and physical properties with the general plasma membrane. Junctional and nonjunctional membranes have a characteristic trilaminar unit membrane appearance in thin sections (the outer leaflets of occludens appear as a single electron dense zone) and an interior fracture plane (1,5,37-40), indicating that hydrophobic domains exist within the junctional membranes (40).

The basis for the linked reaction of various types of cell junctions to tumorigenesis is unknown but several mechanisms seem possible. These include: 1- the absence or defective production of specific junctional components; 2- impediment of junctional assembly mechanisms by changes in the properties of the nonjunctional cell membrane or; 3- impairment of cell-to-cell recognition that may be required for the initiation of symmetrical junction formation. The simultaneous appearance of deficiencies of several types of junctions in carcinomas of the cervix may argue against a defect in the synthesis of junctional components. The second possibility receives support from other observations in the literature. Many membrane alterations accompany the process of malignant transformation and basic structural defects in the composition and/or organization of the general plasma membrane may represent a common denominator to account for these changes (41). A crucial alteration in the general plasma membrane may represent the proximal event resulting in defects in several types of cell junctions. Membrane changes could either be intrinsic or extrinsic. Intrinsic changes (41) that produce an altered microenvironment within the membrane might result in the impediment of assembly of specific junctional components into the nonjunctional membrane. Extrinsic

changes such as modification (42) or increases
(43) of surface polysaccharides would impair
cell-to-cell contact and/or recognition thereby
preventing junction formation. These possibilities are currently under investigation in this
laboratory.

REFERENCES

(1)   N.S. McNutt and R.S. Weinstein, Prog.
      Biophys. Mol. Biol., 26 (1973) 45.

(2)   M.G. Farquhar and G.E. Palade, J. Cell Biol.,
      17 (1963) 375.

(3)   W.R. Loewenstein, Ann. N.Y. Acad. Sci., 137
      (1966) 441.

(4)   B.W. Payton, M.V.L. Bennett and G.D. Pappas,
      Science, 166 (1969) 1641.

(5)   N.S. McNutt and R.S. Weinstein, J. Cell
      Biol., 47 (1970) 666.

(6)   G.D. Pappas, Y. Asada and M.V.L. Bennett,
      J. Cell Biol., 49 (1971) 173.

(7)   M.S. Steinberg, Science, 141 (1963) 401.

(8)   W.R. Loewenstein, Perspectives Biol. Med.,
      11 (1968) 260.

(9)   D.R. Coman, Cancer Res., 13 (1953) 397.

(10) M. Abercrombie and E.J. Ambrose, Cancer
      Res., 22 (1962) 525.

(11) A. Jamanoskosmanovic and W.R. Loewenstein,
      J. Cell Biol., 38 (1968) 556.

(12) J.D. Sheridan, J. Cell Biol., 45 (1970) 91.

(13) P. Emmelot and E.L. Benedetti, in: Carci-
      nogenesis: A Broad Critique, ed. R.W.
      Comley (Williams and Wilkins, Baltimore,
      1967) p. 471.

(14) N.S. McNutt and R.S. Weinstein, Science,
      165 (1969) 597.

(15) N.S. McNutt, R.A. Hershberg and R.S.
      Weinstein, J. Cell Biol., 51 (1971) 805.

(16) A. Martinez-Palomo, Lab. Invest., 22 (1970)
      605.

(17) E. Farber, Cancer Res., 33 (1973) 2537.

(18) H.A. Battifora, R. Eisenstein, H. Sky-Peck
      and J.H. McDonald, J. Urol., 93 (1965) 217.

(19) D.C. Utz, K. Hanash and G.M. Farrow, J.
      Urol., 103 (1970) 160.

(20) M.G. Farquhar and G.E. Palade, J. Cell
      Biol., 26 (1965) 263.

(21) H. Moor and K. Mühlethaler, J. Cell Biol.,
      17 (1963) 609.

(22) F.K. Mostofi, J.A.M.A. 206 (1968) 1764.

(23) H.J. Jewett, in: Urology, Vol. 2 (3rd
      Edition), eds. M.F. Campbell and J.H.
      Harrison (W.B. Saunders Co., Philadelphia,
      1970) p. 1027.

(24) H. Jewett and G.H. Strong, J. Urol., 55
      (1946) 366.

(25) L.D. Johnson, Obstet Gyneco. Surg., 24
      (1969) 735.

(26) L.G. Koss, Lab. Invest., 21 (1969) 154.

(27) G.J. Turnbull, Invest. Urol., 11 (1973)198.

(28) J.B. Wade, J.P. Revel and V.A. DiScala, Am. J. Physiol., 224 (1973) 407.

(29) W.R. Richter and S.M. Moize, J. Ultrastructure Res., 9 (1963) 1.

(30) H. Battifora, R. Eisenstein and J.H. McDonald, Invest. Urol., 1 (1964) 354.

(31) W.R. Loewenstein, S.J. Socolar, S. Higashino, Y. Kanno and N. Davidson, Science, 149 (1965) 295.

(32) M.J. Fulker, E.H. Cooper and T. Tanaka, Cancer, 27 (1971) 71.

(33) E.H. Cooper, Ann. Roy. Coll. Surg. Engl., 51 (1972) 1.

(34) J. Overton, Develop. Biol., 4 (1962) 532.

(35) D.E. Kelly, J. Cell Biol., 28 (1966) 51.

(36) W.S. Krawczyk and G.F. Wilgram, J. Ultrastructure Res., 45 (1973) 93.

(37) J.P. Chalcroft and S. Bullivant, J. Cell Biol., 47 (1970) 49.

(38) N.B. Gilula, D. Branton and P. Satir, Proc. Nat. Acad. Sci., U.S.A., 67 (1970) 213.

(39) L.A. Staehelin, J. Cell Sci., 13 (1974) 763.

(40) D. Branton, Proc. Nat. Acad. Sci., U.S.A., 55 (1966) 1048.

(41) D.F.H. Wallach, Proc. Nat. Acad. Sci., U.S.A., 61 (1968) 868.

(42) C.G. Gahmberg and S.I. Hakomori, Proc. Nat. Acad. Sci., U.S.A., 70 (1973) 3329.

(43)   A. Martinez-Palomo, C. Braislovsky and W. Bernhard, Cancer Res., 29 (1969) 925.

ACKNOWLEDGEMENTS

The authors gratefully acknowledge Mrs. Sharon Zel for assistance in preparing the manuscript. This study was supported by National Cancer Institute Grant CA-14447 from the National Institutes of Health, United States Public Health Service.

DISCUSSION

P. A. Srere, Veterans Administration Hospital: May
I ask you to speculate in terms of what you know about the
structure of the junction and in terms of what the pictures
of a membrane we have been given up to time? For example,
proteins which have centrally hydrophobic regions all the
way through the membrane could not be expected to have a
hydrophilic region through it. Am I extending both lines
of data too far?

R. S. Weinstein, Tufts University: There is little
hard data that is available on the chemical composition
of the intramembranous particles or "subunits" at nexus
junctions, although indirect biochemical evidence suggests
that they are proteins. If asked to speculate, and that's
an invitation that is difficult to turn down, I would
suggest that the particles viewed in freeze-cleave preparations of nexus membranes represent "cylindrical"
proteins that are oriented with their long axis perpendicular to the plane of the membrane. The segment of the
cylinder that is intercalated within the membrane may have
a hydrophobic exterior. An interior hydrophilic pore
may span the length of the cylinder and provide a channel
for the direct transfer of molecules from cell to cell
(NcNutt and Weinstein, J. Cell Biol. 47 [1970] 666).

P. A. Srere: Both those things seem to be
inconsistent with each other. You have to have a protein
that has a water hole through it, whereas the amino acid
composition would indicate a structure that would exclude
such a water hole. I wonder also if anyone has calulated
what the radius of rotation of the fluorescein molecule
would be, is it sufficiently small to fit through a
protein whose diameter is about 90 Å?

W. R. Loewenstein, Univeristy of Miami: I don't
recall the precise equivalent hydrodynamic diameter, but

I think it probably fits if the channel is an aqueous one.

W. S. Lynn, Duke Medical Center: We have heard a lot about proteases and various glycosidases which remove part of the fuzz from the suface of the membrane. Is there any quantitative data to make any correlation at all between this fuzz and the junctions which might contain components of this fuzz?

R. S. Weinstein: It has been suggested that excessively thick surface coats may block the formation of some types of cell junctions (Martinez-Palomo, et al., Cancer Res. 29 [1969] 925). Also, Orci and his associates have examined the effects of a proteolytic enzyme, that may remove surface materials, on junction formation (Orci et al., Science 180 [1973] 647). They exposed isolated pancreatic islet cells to very low concentrations of pronase and were able to induce the formation of extensive occludens junctions. These findings seem to point to a relationship between surface coats and the production of junctions.

W. S. Lynn: Yes.

I. Fritz, University of Toronto: I have a question along that same line. Would you please comment about the turnover of these junctions. What determines the rates of formation and dissociation of various types of junctions, and what factors influence these rates?

R. S. Weinstein: Fully functional nexus junctions can form very rapidly, probably in a matter of minutes. This has been elegantly demonstrated by Ito and Loewenstein (Devel. Biol. 19 [1969] 228). Desmosomes (maculae adherentes) are assembled at a more leisurely rate and apparently require hours to reach the final stage in their morphogenesis. I suspect that occludens junctions (e.g., tight junctions) form quite rapidly.

I. Fritz: I was impressed by the observations of Goodenough that tight junctions are broken rapidly in hypertonic media. In the reformation of tight junctions, is there any evidence that new protein synthesis is required? Or is the dissociation-reassociation independent of synthetic processes?

R. S. Weinstein: To the best of my knowledge, the point has not been experimentally determined.

H. G. Hempling, Medical University of South Carolina: This is for Dr. Loewenstein, perhaps some tumor cells have electrophysiological properties different from control cells. Have you had an occasion to fuse cells of different electrophysiological properties and if so what happens to the electrophysiological properties of the hybrid.

W. R. Loewenstein: What electrophysiological properties are you referring to?

H. G. Hempling: Specifically membrane potential and perhaps membrane resistance.

W. R. Loewenstein: Nonjunctional or junctional ones?

H. G. Hempling: Really it makes no difference as long as they have different electrophysiological properties. I am curious to know whether when you fuse the hybrids whether the membrane characteristics fuse? Or whether the electrophysiological properties assume those of one or the other type of cell?

W. R. Loewenstein: We have looked only at junctional properties; these are the ones I spoke about. We have not been interested in nonjunctional membrane properties. I should like to add just one more point of information about junctions in answer to the question raised by someone at the other side of the hall. One can make junctions in vitro in appropriate cell system. Ito and I have used giant cells from early newt embryos. We start with separate cells and then manipulate them together at well defined spots of their membranes. It takes on the average 4-10 min. for the cells to make communicating junctions under such experimental conditions. If we now pull the cells apart by micromanipulation and then bring them together at other spots, it takes again 4-10 min. to make a communicating junction. However, if the cells are brought together at the same spot, full junction formation takes place within less than 3 sec. Junctional formation is

markedly facilitated in a membrane region which has previously contained a communicating junction (S. Ito, E. Sato
& W. R. Loewenstein, J. Membrane Biol., in press).

L. Warren, University of Pennsylvania: One little
question of my own. Do you have any feeling for the relative number of junctions that exist between cells that are
in growth phase and those in a plateau phase of growth? I
say that because, if it is true that the turnover of the
surface membrane of cells in plateau phases is higher than
that in a growth phase then you might think that the
rejection of membranes during turnover would lead to a
rather unstable situation with the possible breakage of
junction.

R. S. Weinstein: It is well known that some types
of junctions persist throughout the mitotic cycle. However, junctional frequencies have not been examined at
various points in the cell cycle nor have they been
correlated with growth phase.

L. Warren: One could predict on certain grounds that
there would be more, when there was less turnover with a
more static membrane.

SOME METABOLIC EFFECTS OF ENVIRONMENTAL pH ON
NORMAL AND CANCER CELLS

H. EAGLE
Department of Cell Biology
Albert Einstein College of Medicine

Abstract: The growth and metabolism of cultured mammalian
cells are profoundly modified by the environmental pH.
At the optimum pH, which varies from pH 6.8 - 7.8 in
individual strains (4), cells grow more rapidly and
attain higher population densities (2)(3)(5). The optimum pH for the synthesis of globulin by mouse myeloma
cells, and of collagen by human, mouse or rat fibroblasts (7), coincided with that for cellular growth.
However, the optimum pH for the synthesis of S 100 protein by rat astrocytes (pH 6.4 - 6.8) was significantly
more acid than that for cellular growth (7.15 - 7.8)
(8).

The synthesis of reovirus by mouse and rat cells
was markedly pH-dependent, with a sharply-defined optimum at pH 7.2 which did not coincide with that for
cellular growth (9). Similarly, the optimum pH for the
hybridization of certain mouse and human cells was pH
7.8 - 8.0 (10), significantly more alkaline than that
for cellular growth. The optimum pH for the rescue of
SV40 by the fusion of transformed human or mouse cells
with a permissive monkey line was pH 8.0 - 8.4 (11), a
range ultimately lethal to both parent strains as well
as to their hybrid progeny.

The mechanism of these effects is under continuing study.

INTRODUCTION

When animal cells are cultured in the usual bicarbo-
nate-buffered media, the initial alkalinization due to a
loss of CO_2 to the atmosphere is followed by a progressive
acidification at a rate and to a degree which depends on
the cell number and the metabolic activity of the specific
strain (Fig. 1). Those pH shifts are significantly reduced but not entirely eliminated when the cells are grown
in vessels exposed to a 5-10% CO_2 atmosphere, rather than
in a stoppered container. The addition to the medium of
non-volatile organic buffers, selected on the basis of
toxicity from those synthesized by Good et al. (Table 1),
greatly reduces that pH variation, and has permitted a sys-
tematic inquiry into the effects of environmental pH on
cellular growth, metabolism and function. The present
paper summarizes the significant and in some instances
striking effects of environmental pH on a) cellular growth;
b) the synthesis of specialized proteins (globulin, collagen and S 100 protein); c) the synthesis of reovirus;
d) the efficiency of cellular fusion and hybridization;
and e) the efficiency of SV40 virus rescue.

RESULTS AND DISCUSSION

A. Cellular growth and contact inhibition

Both the rate of cellular multiplication, and the
maximum population ultimately attained, have proved
markedly pH-dependent (2)(3) (Fig. 2), the optimum pH
varying from strain to strain in the range pH 6.8 - 7.8
(4). With some strains there was a sharply defined optimum; with others, there was a broad zone within which pH
variation had relatively little effect. The degree of
variation in the optimal pH of cell strains from a single
animal species is illustrated for rat cells in Fig. 3.

At that optimum, some strains attain maximum population densities as much as 3-5 times greater than those in
unbuffered* cultures. This has important implications

---

*i.e., containing only bicarbonate as the buffering agent

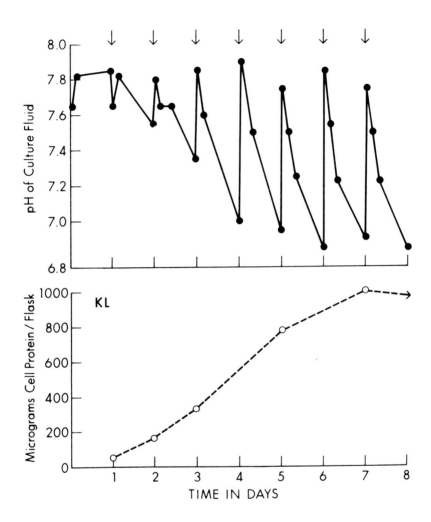

Fig. 1. pH variation in a human fibroblast (KL) culture
buffered with 24 mM NaHCO$_3$ (from Eagle (1)).

TABLE 1

Buffer Concentrations (mM) Recommended for Media at Indicated pH [a,b]

Buffers	pKa	6.4	6.6	6.8	7.0	7.2	7.4	7.6	7.8	8.0	8.2	8.4	8.6	For general use[c]
BIS TRIS	6.46	10												
PIPES	6.8	10	10	10	10									
BES	7.15		10	15	10	15	10	10						10
TES	7.5						10	10	15	10				
HEPES	7.55				10	10	15	15	15	15				15
EPPS	8.0									10	15	10		10
TRICINE	8.15										15	15	15	
BICINE	8.35											10	15	
Na$_2$HPO$_4$	6.7	10	10	10	2	-	-	-	-	-	-	-	-	
NaHCO$_3$[d]		0.5	0.5	1	2	5	10	15	20	30	40	60	80[e]	15

(a) Concentrations of organic buffers to be halved if toxicity is noted for specific cell line, and to be halved also for primary cultures, direct from tissues.

(b) Conveniently added as 1% of 1 M stock solution (PIPES at 500 mM). Most of these buffers are strongly acidic or basic, and medium must be adjusted to desired pH with NaOH or HCl.

(c) Although this buffer combination is moderately effective over the pH range 7.0 - 8.0, the pH fluctuations will be somewhat greater than with the combinations suggested for a specific pH range.

(d) Concentrations which provide indicated pH (approximately) in open containers (Petri dishes) in CO$_2$ incubator with 2-5% CO$_2$ atmosphere. Bicarbonate concentration may be kept at 15 mM for stoppered containers.

(e) Upper safe limits in terms of total osmolarity.

154

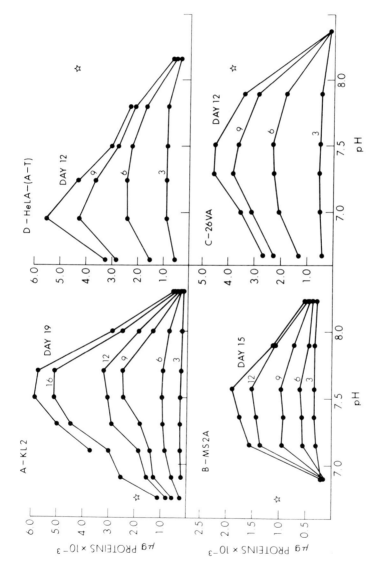

Fig. 2. The growth of human cells as a function of the medium pH (Ceccarini and Eagle (2)).

155

RAT

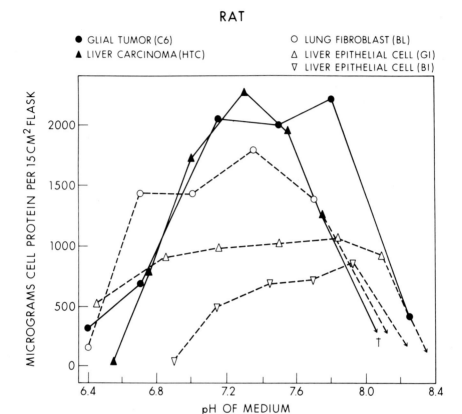

● GLIAL TUMOR (C6)   ○ LUNG FIBROBLAST (BL)
▲ LIVER CARCINOMA (HTC)   △ LIVER EPITHELIAL CELL (GI)
                            ▽ LIVER EPITHELIAL CELL (BI)

Legend to Fig. 3. The growth of rat cells as a function of medium pH. The ordinates indicate the micrograms of cell protein per 15 cm^2 flask after 6 - 8 days, with an inoculum of 6 - 12 x 10^5 cells.

with respect to the phenomenon of "contact"-inhibition, i.e., the almost complete cessation of growth in normal cell cultures at relatively low population densities, presumably triggered by cellular contact. Growth could be re-initiated in stabilized ("contact"-inhibited) cultures in unbuffered media merely by changing the pH to the optimum level for that specific strain; conversely, growth was abruptly terminated in cultures growing at the optimal pH if the buffer was removed (5) (Fig. 4). Clearly, contact as such is not the sole determinant of growth arrest in crowded cultures, and may not be even a primary factor. Rather, there appears to be a population-dependent inhibition of growth (6). The absolute level at which the population density stabilizes varies from strain to strain, varies with the serum concentration in the medium, and is pH-dependent.

In appropriately buffered media, and with frequent changes of media, the differences between normal and malignant cells with respect to maximum population density are reduced, but do not altogether disappear. Cancer cells and virus transformants tend to grow somewhat faster, and usually achieve a somewhat higher population density. In addition, most normal cells in stabilized cultures, if adequately re-fed, remain viable for days and weeks, while the generality of cancer cells and virus transformants tend to become necrotic, or to slough off the glass or plastic substrate in coherent sheets.

B. Synthesis of specialized proteins

It was to have been anticipated that the pH optimum for the synthesis of some specialized proteins would be essentially the same as those for the growth and multiplication of the cell itself. This has proved to be the case for the synthesis of globulin by mouse myeloma cells (Scharff and Eagle, unpublished observations) and of collagen by mouse, human and rat fibroblasts (7). In contrast, however, the accumulation of S 100 protein within a rat astrocyte had a well-defined optimum in the range of pH 6.4 - 6.8, significantly more acid than the pH optimal for the growth of the cell (8).

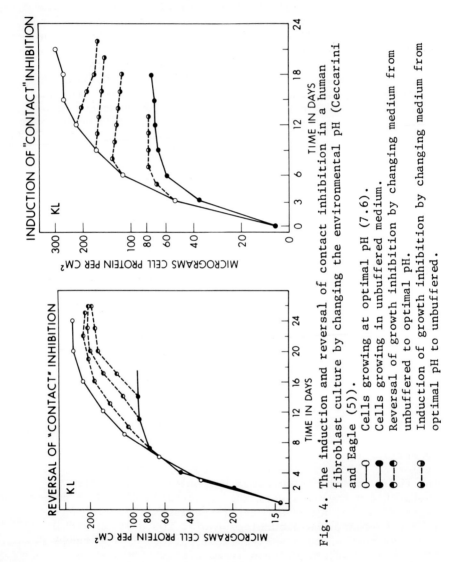

Fig. 4. The induction and reversal of contact inhibition in a human fibroblast culture by changing the environmental pH (Ceccarini and Eagle (5)).

○——○ Cells growing at optimal pH (7.6).

●——● Cells growing in unbuffered medium.

◑——◑ Reversal of growth inhibition by changing medium from unbuffered to optimal pH.

◑——◑ Induction of growth inhibition by changing medium from optimal pH to unbuffered.

158

C. The synthesis of reovirus by mouse and rat cells

The L929 mouse cell grows well over a broad pH range (7.0 - 7.8), and an epithelial cell culture from adult rat liver has a well-defined growth optimum at pH 7.8 (4). In both cases, however, the optimum pH for reovirus synthesis was pH 7.2 (9) (Fig. 5). The sharpness of the curve relating virus yield to environmental pH is particularly to be noted. In some experiments a shift in environmental pH of only 0.4 pH units was associated with as much as a 10-fold decrease in virus yield.

D. Cellular fusion and hybridization

Environmental pH had a modest effect on the efficiency of cellular fusion by e.g. Sendai virus, and a far more significant effect on the subsequent hybridization, i.e., the fusion of the two nuclei in the heterokaryon into a single nucleus, with the formation of a viable hybrid cell. In the cell systems so far studied, the optimum pH for both fusion and hybridization was significantly more alkaline than that optimal for the growth of either parent or of the hybrid progeny. The percentage of cell fusions increased 3 to 5-fold at pH 8.0 as compared with pH 7.2, while the yield of hybrid colonies increased in some experiments as much as 100-fold (10) (Fig. 6). The optimum pH for the hybridization of a number of cell types with widely varying pH optima for growth, is under current examination.

The pH-sensitive step in cellular hybridization occurs during the first 4-6 days after cellular fusion. The yield of hybrid colonies increased with the time for which they were kept at pH 8.0 over the first 4-6 days; conversely, the yield decreased progressively in relation to the time at which the cells were kept at pH 7.2, before being shifted upward to the pH optimal for hybridization (Fig. 7). The nature of this pH-sensitive step is under continuing study.

159

Legend to Fig. 5.   The effect of environmental pH on reovirus synthesis (●—●) and cellular
growth (O--O) in an epithelial rat
liver cell (Fields and Eagle (6)).

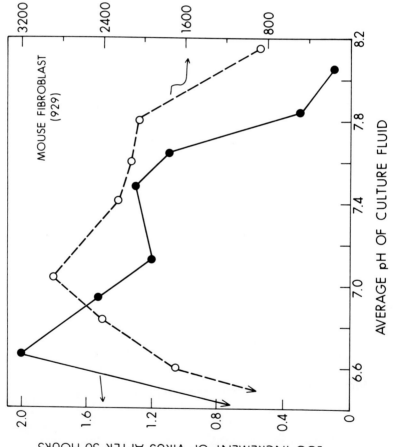

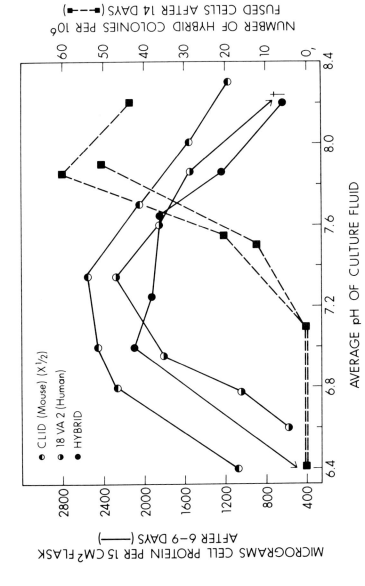

Fig. 6. The effect of environmental pH on the hybrid-ization of mouse and human cell (Croce et al., (10)).

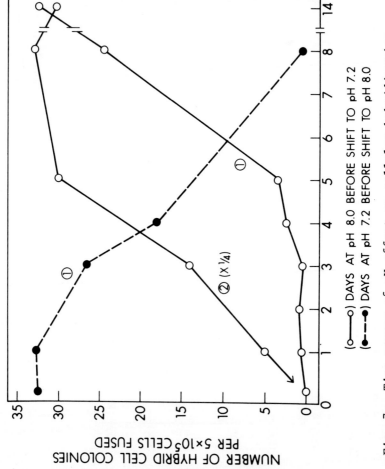

Fig. 7. Time course of pH effect on cellular hybridization (Croce, Koprowski and Eagle (10)).

(o——o) DAYS AT pH 8.0 BEFORE SHIFT TO pH 7.2
(●——●) DAYS AT pH 7.2 BEFORE SHIFT TO pH 8.0

NUMBER OF HYBRID CELL COLONIES PER 5×10⁵ CELLS FUSED

E. Virus rescue

The intact SV40 viral genome is present in virus transformants, evidenced by the continuing synthesis of virus-specific proteins, and more conclusively by the fact that complete virus is synthesized (rescued) if the transformed cells are fused with an appropriate permissive strain. The rescue of SV40 virus from transformed mouse or human cells on fusion with permissive monkey cells was extraordinarily pH-sensitive, with an increase of 2-4 logs in the titer of virus rescued after seven days when the pH of the medium was increased from e.g. 6.8 to 8.4 (11). It is to be noted that the pH optimal for virus rescue in these experiments was ultimately lethal to both parental cells, as well as the hybrid progeny. As in the case of hybridization, the pH-sensitive process determining the ultimate yield of virus took place in the first four days after cellular fusion (Fig. 8). By that time, cells kept at pH 8 were already programmed ultimately to produce SV40 virus in high titer. Studies are in progress to determine whether the same underlying process may be responsible for the high pH optimum for cellular hybridization (7.8 - 8.0) and virus rescue (8.0 - 8.4). The apparent difference in the optimal pH may simply reflect the fact that cellular hybridization necessarily involves the continuing multiplication of the cell, while virus rescue is a short-term process which could occur in a cell which would actually not survive the alkaline pH optimal for viral synthesis.

The effect on virus rescue of environmental factors other than pH is under continuing study. The possibility may be considered that under optimal conditions, in which the efficiency of virus rescue from known transformants is increased by 2-4 logs, viruses may be rescued from cells in which their presence is suspected but not yet demonstrated.

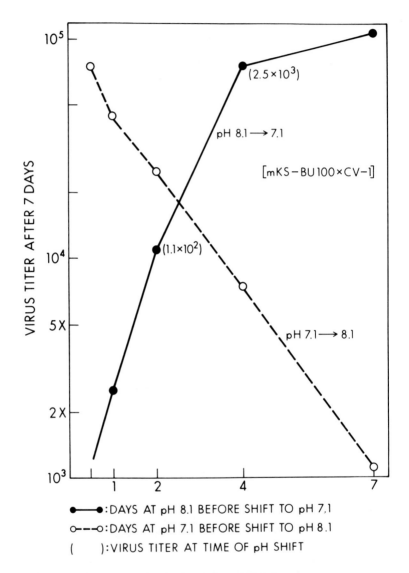

Fig. 8. The time course of SV40 synthesis at pH 7.1 and 8.2 in SV40 transformants fused with a permissive monkey cell (Croce, Koprowski and Eagle (unpublished).

REFERENCES

(1) Eagle, H., Science 174 (1971) 500.

(2) Ceccarini, C. and Eagle, H., Proc. Natl. Acad. Sci. 68 (1971) 229.

(3) Rubin, H., J. Cell Biol. (1971) 686.

(4) Eagle, H., J. Cell. Physiol. 82 (1973) 82.

(5) Ceccarini, C. and Eagle, H., Nature New Biology 233 (1971) 271.

(6) Stoker, M.G.P. and Rubin, H., Nature 215 (1967) 171.

(7) Nigra, T.P., Martin, G.H. and Eagle, H., Biochem. Biophys. Res. Comm. 53 (1973) 272.

(8) Pfeiffer, S. and Eagle, H., In preparation.

(9) Fields, B.N. and Eagle, H., Virology 52 (1973) 581.

(10) Croce, C.M., Koprowski, H. and Eagle, H., Proc. Natl. Acad. Sci. 69 (1972) 1953.

(11) Calothy, G., Croce, C.M., Defendi, V., Koprowski, H. and Eagle, H., Proc. Natl. Acad. Sci. 70 (1973) 366.

DISCUSSION

W. R. Loewenstein, University of Miami: I'd like to start off the discussion by making a comment on your fusion experiment. There is an interesting parallel here between the pH effects on cell fusion and those on junction formation. In myoblast fusion -- this is a membrane fusion occurring naturally during embryogenesis, not a fusion provoked by Sendai virus --Douglas Fambrough has shown that, preceding the actual membrane fusion, there is an intermediate step of gap junction formation. Now, we know also that in a junctional communication the pH of the medium is important. Junctional communication is interfered with a low pH.

H. Eagle, Albert Einstein College of Medicine: Which pH specifically?

W. R. Loewenstein: If I remember well the data Nakas, Socolar, and I got some time ago, pH below 6 impaired communication. There is no impairment on the alkaline side up to about pH 10 (J. gen. Physiol. $\underline{50}$:1065-1891, 1967).

J. Roth, Biocenter: I'd like to report two observations and maybe some questions will be raised. The first observation is an increase in protein export by normal cells as they approach confluence. I noticed that many of the graphs you used involved the cell protein per flask as opposed to cell number; even though the cells will reach confluence, they will keep on producing protein and I assumed that this would be accounted for in your calculations.

H. Eagle: We routinely plotted cell protein in the figures shown, but the relationships are essentially the same if the data are plotted in terms of cell number, rather than protein.

J. Roth: The other observation related to pH, which I certainly hope isn't anachronistic, is that we studied the effects of pH on amino acid binding to serum proteins in Dulbecco's modified medium and we found that there is definitely a change in many amino acids in their binding to serum between the pH of physiological growth between 6.8 and pH 8. There were changes in both directions, as the media went from basic to acidic some of the amino acids were more tightly bound and some of them were more losely bound.

H. Eagle: When you refer to binding, do you mean such things as the linkage of cysteine to protein - SH groups?

J. Roth: No specific binding of amino acids to serum proteins, not specific binding, not any kind of co-valent binding.

. *R. Longton, Naval Medical Research Institute:* Is your phenomenon of cell senessence (senility) similar to increased numbers of serial passages of cells from a cell line?

H. Eagle: One can express the age of the culture either in terms of the number of culture passages or the number of cell doublings. I think the more significant number is the number of cell doublings.

R. Longton: Well, we found this to be a problem in trying to attain primary cultures. We found if we added millipore filtered cell exposed media from earlier generations to older generations, we could increase the number of serial passages. This was a factor we felt could be important in senessence. The factor at this point is not identified, but we are able to get an increased number of serial passages through the factors acquired from earlier generations.

H. Eagle: I was just going to ask you what you think is going on here.

G. Koch, Roche Institute of Molecular Biology: It might be of interest to mention that Dr. B. Boenicke (1961, Thesis, University of Hamburg, Germany) in my laboratory several years ago studied the effect of pH and cell density on the replication of poliovirus in cells grown in suspension. The pH was kept constant by a pH stat, that is automatically by addition of base. The yield of poliovirus/cell was found to be independent of the pH between 6.9 and 8.2 and of the cell concentration between 5×10^5 and 1×10^7 cell/ml, but the virus yield per cell decreased sharply below and above these pH values and when the cell density was raised above 1×10^7/ml.

M. Lubin, Dartmouth Medical School: I want to preface my question by noting that year after year Dr. Eagle comes up with an assortment of phenomena that sets us all back on our heels, and those of us who work with tissue culture just are astonished to think why didn't the rest of us come up with this simple approach ourselves, so we're all in debt to Dr. Eagle for continuing to clarify so many problems in the field of tissue culture. My question is this, all of the phenomena you described are those involving synthesis of macromolecules, virus production, DNA synthesis, and so forth. Have you had a chance to look at the pH optima of those processes which involve just membrane binding, for example lectin agglutination?

H. Eagle: No, we have not. I have been discussing with Paul Atkinson and Stan Nathenson some exploratory experiments to determine the effects of environmental pH on membrane structure. These will be undertaken in the near future, unless some of you have already done it.

V. P. Hollander, Hospital for Joint Diseases: Dr. Eagle, you referred to intracellular pH as a possible factor. Could you speculate on how one could approach the concept that the difference in ultimate cell density between transformed and normal cells may be a function? My second question has to do with your measurements of synthesis of macromolecules in culture from incorporation of small radioactive precursors. Do you think such a procedure is valid when you vary pH over wide range and probably change intracellular pool size?

H. Eagle: That's a good question. We have indeed looked at the specific activity of the overall intracellular pool as a function of pH, and have found no differences.

L. Warren, University of Pennsylvania: As for pH studies that you just mentioned, we have checked the profiles of the glycopeptides of cells growing in hepes buffer, various buffers, and we didn't find anything of particular interest. There wasn't much variation. A second point, yesterday after I spoke, Dr. MacPherson asked a question about the plateau phase of transformed cells, C 13/B4. I think his implication was how could you get that because transformed cells just don't plateau, their numbers go up and then they go down. He drew a picture of the growth curve and so do you. You have shown those beautiful growth curves on a slide, but the fact is that the flat part of the curve is from 4 to 8 days long before they start petering and the curve declines. This is a long time, certainly adequate to do all sorts of experiments on the plateau state. The question I'd like to ask is what importance do you ascribe to the fact that the control cells stop growing and the transformed cells keep growing slowly for 8 days and then the curve declines. Is there anything fundamental there that you can see?

H. Eagle: We are still in the phenomenologic stage, in that the observations are as yet unexplained. As somebody once said, the words "always" and "never" should never be used in biology, and this is true here also. Although in general, malignant cells show the behaviour shown in one of my slides, and which Dr. Macpherson also referred to yesterday, there are some transformants which in this respect (plateau phenomenon) behave like normal cells.

L. Warren: But with all these transformed cells, you work with, and they are pretty standard type cells, there is a 4 to 8 day plateau. Wouldn't you call that "plateau"?

H. Eagle: It's a plateau in terms of cell protein or cell number. I would be reluctant to work with a culture of virus-transformed or cancer cells 6 - 8 days after they has attained a saturation (plateau) level. If you clone such cultures to determine the percentage of viable cells, one usually finds this is going steadily downhill.

I. MacPherson, Imperial Cancer Research Fund Laboratories: I think you can sometimes get a false plateau with transformed cells where there's a balance between new cell growth and cell death and this can persist for quite some time.

L. Warren: If you pulse these with tritiated thymidine you may get a somewhat enhanced incorporation, but it isn't all that much over that of control cells. That plateau is not caused by a balance of ferocious division and ferocious dying, it's essentially the same. There may be some important difference, but you can't see it.

H. Eagle: I think it's quite possible that in such plateaued and dying cultures, one might find no important difference in the structure of a cell membrane over 3- or 4-day period.

W. Lands, University of Michigan: I also wanted to ask a question about the death process. A lot of attention is paid to growth (I suppose it's our youth oriented culture) but death is not a particularly popular event. As you said, the normal cells can hang on for a long time. At the phenomenological level, can you mix normal and transformed cells in different percentages and then look at the die-away curves? Can you see whether there's an environmental effect of one cell on another on the death process? It might help to understand whether it's an internal or externalized event. Have you tried anything like that?

H. Eagle: Only in the sense that if you do this, make this mixed culture, the transformed cell usually overgrows the normal cell.

W. Lands: If you do it under conditions where they should be at the plateau though, then it shouldn't be overgrowing, and then the question is: would the cells remain stationery?

H. Eagle: We haven't done the experiment.

B. B. Lavietes, New York University Medical Center:
In a situation where a specific protein is synthesized
by a normal cell and its transformed analog, is there a
shift in the pH optimum for that specific protein's
synthesis?

H. Eagle: If you mean the same protein being
synthesized by a normal and transformed cell, no, we
haven't looked at that. The closest we've come to that
experiment is to look at collagen synthesis by 3 cell
lines in which the optimum pH for the growth of the cell
varied from 7.2 to 7.8. In each case the optimum pH
for the synthesis of collagen was the same as that for
the growth for the specific cell line.

Z. Brada, Papanicolaou Cancer Research Institute:
Dr. Eagle, can you comment on the problem of contact
inhibition of movement?

H. Eagle: There is a clear dissociation between
these two phenomena. I don't think anything I've said
is applicable directly without experiment to the phenomenon
of cell movement.

J. Kowal, University Hospitals: I think the
problems you described relating to the enviromental
conditions are well taken. In our own work with adrenal
culture cells, we found profound effects of pH on rate of
lactic acid synthesis from glucose, cyclic-AMP turnover,
and steroid synthesis. Raising the pH just a half pH
unit can result in a doubling or tripling in the rate of
glycolysis. Unless one has carefully controlled these
conditions you can produce a variety of effects that may
not be real.

S. Roseman, Johns Hopkins University: I'm going to
ask an utterly naive question. Have you looked or thought
about the effect of the microenvironment, that is the
environment around the cell? In particular when cells
come into what we call confluence is it true that the
layer beneath the cell surface, between the cells and
the glass is truly in equilibrium with the supernatant
fluid? Do you know the answer to this question?

H. Eagle: No.

S. Roseman: Since they're pouring out a lot of acid at that time, is it possible that the pH below the cell in fact is not quite the same as the pH above the cell?

H. Eagle: It's quite possible. Your comment makes me think it might be worthwhile to do some critical experiments in media in which the galactose or a combination of pyruvate and ribose is used instead of glucose. Glycolysis is then fractional as compared to that in glucose medium.

S. Roseman: Actually, I think it could be done these days with fluorescent pH indicators or something which might be trapped.

H. Eagle: Have you reason to believe that when a cell is adhering to a surface of plastic or glass, there is a fluid layer beneath the cell?

S. Roseman: Well at the last Gordon Conference there was a lot of discussion about work in this area and its very clear from some beautiful pictures presented there that you don't have a rim of the cell as I once thought, but it just touches down, the cell touches down in a few points, perhaps 3 or 4, at the leading edge by the way, at the ruffling membrane. So you would think then that when the cell is moving around, the medium on top is in equilibrium with the solution beneath, but I'm not so sure. Perhaps the people working on electrical junctions can tell us whether cells in the confluent layer are in true equilibrium with the solution above.

REGULATION OF GROWTH IN ANIMAL CELLS

H. RUBIN
Department of Molecular Biology
University of California, Berkeley

Abstract: The multiplication of animal cells in culture
     can be stimulated by a variety of unrelated sub-
     stances.   It appears that the cell is a poised system,
     and that non-lethal or sub-lethal perturbations in its
     outer membrane will initiate a programmed series of
     events leading to increased metabolism and multi-
     plication.   These perturbations initiate a set of
     diverse processes, including changes in permeability,
     energy metabolism and biosynthesis.   At least some of
     these processes are independent of one another
     although several are required to initiate DNA syn-
     thesis.   All changes produced by "biological"
     effectors such as serum, population density and virus
     transformation can be simulated by pH.   It is propos-
     ed that intracellular pH is the mediating cellular
     variable which controls the diverse processes.   A
     simple model for pH control based on the anionic
     permeability of the membrane is presented.

INTRODUCTION

     Compensatory growth in the organism may occur in res-
ponse to local or systemic stimuli.   The prototype of the
local stimulus is the phenomenon of wound healing, while
that of the systemic is liver regeneration (1).   Wound
healing occurs in one form or another in every tissue of
the body, but it has been most thoroughly studied in
easily accessible tissues such as epidermis and tongue.
In general, the generative basal cells of the intact

173

epithelium grow at a slow rate, replacing those of the
more superficial layers which have been removed. When
wounding occurs, i.e.: a discontinuity is created--the
cells adjacent to the wound respond by migrating and multi-
plying at an increased rate until the damaged tissue has
been replaced.

When a major portion of the liver is removed, the
compensatory growth is not restricted to the region of the
incision but occurs throughout the remaining tissue.
Again it ceases when the functional tissue is replaced.

In both cases compensatory growth appears to be
superimposed upon day to day physiological mechanisms
which control the growth rates of the cells. While much
has been learned about compensatory growth in the whole
organism, the experimental systems have been too complex
and unmanipulable to yield any conclusive knowledge about
the mechanism of cellular growth control. It is toward
this end that experiments on growth control in tissue
culture have been directed.

The basic phenomenon in tissue culture which has
served as the focus of interest has been variously called
contact inhibition (2), density dependent inhibition (3)
or topoinhibition (4). I shall use the term density
dependent inhibition for reasons explained some six years
ago (3). The term refers to the fact that the growth rate
of cultured cells decreases as their population density
increases. The most pronounced change in growth rate
occurs at about the time the cell sheet becomes confluent
and results in the so-called monolayering tendency of
cells. Unfortunately, the terminology is misleading.
There is no indication that contact itself is a significant inhibitor of growth among normal cells. Indeed, contact enhances the growth of some. Nor does growth cease
with normal cells upon confluency (5). This erroneous
impression has been furthered by emphasis on a highly abnormal line of cells called 3T3 which have been selected
for an exaggerated dependency on population density. The
growth rate of normal cells decreases when they reach confluency, but they go on growing at the reduced rate. This
leads to the false impression of a "saturation density"
when the cells may be continuously increasing in number (6).

A great multiplicity of findings has been reported about the factors involved in growth regulation in tissue culture, but many of them are ignored in the speculation which runs rife in attempts to explain the mechanism of this regulation. Thus, in just a few years we have had chalones, or self-inhibitory macromolecules effusing from cells, altered histones, stimulatory cyclic nucleotides, inhibitory cyclic nucleotides, altered surface receptors, altered permeability to everything, and others in an ever growing list. It is my intention in this analysis to organize the information we have about growth regulation according to various stages of that regulation. After considering the diversity of influences operating at each stage, I shall infer certain generalities about each stage, and attempt to synthesize these into a theoretical mechanism of regulation which embraces all the observations. In my opinion, the collective findings to date can be explained by a unitary mechanism, applicable to all cells. It will be the task for the future to put the theory to further test.

Factors which influence the growth rate of animal cells
in culture

In Table 1, I have listed a selection of factors which affect the growth rate of cells in culture.

TABLE 1

Growth stimulatory for chick embryo cells

A. Physiological
Low population density
Viral transformation
Serum, insulin, proteolytic enzymes
High pH

B. Pathological
Subtoxic Zn,Cd,Mn (not Ca,Mg,Co,Cu,Mo,Ni,Al,Fe)
Dimethylbenzanthracene
(not methylcholanthrene, benzpyrene)

Growth inhibitory
High population density
Absence of serum
Low pH
Deprivation of Zn only
Not dibutyryl cyclic AMP

175

I have omitted those nutritional factors which are essential to growth. Foremost amongst these are the essential amino acids (7). Without them, DNA synthesis cannot be initiated, and cells die. Given a minimal concentration for cell growth, however, the rate of cell growth cannot be influenced by the concentration of amino acids. Cells whose growth has been slowed with increasing population density, cannot be speeded up by increasing the concentration of amino acids (6). Nor can the growth rate of sparse cells be slowed down by decreasing the concentration of amino acids short of that minimal amount required for survival. Thus, though essential, the amino acids are not regulatory.

In a modified sense, the same can be said for glucose (6,7). Here, the absolute requirement for external glucose for the initiation of DNA synthesis in short term experiments is not always demonstrable. The requirement for glucose in such experiments is highly erratic. In general, it can be said that the concentration of glucose can be reduced by a factor of 5 or 10 without affecting the initiation of DNA synthesis in short term experiments. Occasionally glucose can be omitted entirely, but the conditions are not currently controllable. Fibroblasts have reserves of glycogen (8), and energy can also be supplied by amino acids. The important element here is that the rate of supply of glucose cannot be a regulatory event. This needs stressing (see below), since the great variability in the rate of glucose uptake by cells in rough proportion with the growth rate of cells might suggest a causative rather than an associative relationship between glucose utilization and growth rate.

None of the other components ordinarily added to the growth medium effect the growth rate of cells in anything approaching a physiological manner. Special attention, however, needs to be given to zinc, which is not added to the medium deliberately, but which is present in serum and other biological products such as tryptose phosphate broth in relatively high concentrations ($\sim$50 μM/l in chicken serum) and is also present in the distilled water used in making up medium. When zinc is complexed by chelating agents, cells continue to synthesize protein at normal rates, but the initiation of DNA synthesis is blocked (9).

However, the absence of zinc does not affect a number of other properties associated with different growth states (10), and its availability from the medium cannot be considered a regulatory factor. Its availability within the cell, however, might be a significant factor in specific processes leading to DNA synthesis.

The first series of factors in Table 1 may be considered physiological, and includes biological factors such as virus infection, population density and pH which vary in different natural circumstances. Included among these is serum, although there is no indication that its concentration varies in different conditions in vivo. It is merely known that serum is required for cell growth in culture, and that growth rate can be controlled by varying serum concentration. It has been contended that the effect of population density is to alter the surface area accessible to the stimulatory action of serum. If this is to be translated into physiological situations in the organism, such as wound healing, the change in cellular physiognomy would have to be considered the primary variable, with the constant serum concentration serving as the backdrop. In this sense, serum might be considered a nutrient, required for survival were it not for the distinction that added serum can stimulate density inhibited cells to further multiplication.

The best defined way to regulate cell growth is by varying external pH (6,11). Increases of pH up to 8 tend to increase the rate of DNA synthesis, and decreases do the opposite. Within the range of pH 6 to pH 8, the changes are reversible. The effects of pH are strongly dependent on population density of the culture. At high population density, the maximum rate of growth is reached at a pH of about 7.5, while at low population density the maximal rate is reached at a pH of about 7.0, i.e.: it requires about a 3 times higher concentration of protons to inhibit the growth of sparse cells than of crowded cells. The pH sensitivity of crowded cells can be made like that of sparse cells by adding to the crowded cultures a high concentration of serum (12). Malignant cells even when crowded respond to pH as do sparse normal cells.

One simple interpretation of these results is that the pH within sparse, or serum stimulated cells is 0.5 units higher than that of crowded cells. There is ample evidence to indicate that varying external pH of cells in vitro causes changes of internal pH (13). Unfortunately, we have found no satisfactory way of measuring internal pH in monolayer tissue culture. It is possible, however, to erect fairly simple schemes in which the internal pH of cells would vary under different physiological conditions despite constant external pH. These will be considered below.

Table 1 also lists a series of non-physiological stimulators of cell growth. Excessive concentrations of the divalent cations zinc, cadmium and manganese stimulate growth (14). This is particularly evident in the absence of serum, where the basal growth rate is decreased. These metals are effective only at concentrations just below the toxic level. They cannot be used to sustain growth over a long period of time. Other metals which do not produce toxic effects in culture, do not stimulate growth.

The polynuclear hydrocarbon, 9,10 dimethyl-1,2 benz-anthracene (DMBA), perhaps the most potent carcinogen known, also stimulates growth, but stimulatory and toxic manifestations occur at the same concentrations, and it is difficult to demonstrate net increase in cell number (14). Other carcinogenic hydrocarbons, which are not toxic to chicken cells in culture, fail to stimulate growth. (Unfortunately, the relative carcinogenic potential of these compounds in chickens is not established so there is little one can say about the possible relationships between their growth stimulatory and toxic properties, and carcinogenesis).

A variety of other defined materials have been claimed to stimulate cell multiplication. These include proteolytic enzymes (15), digitonin, ribonuclease, hyaluronidase (16) and antibodies to cells (17). Of these, only the first has been extensively tested in the chick embryo system and found to be effective. Whatever the final content of the list of stimulators, it is already inescapable that it includes a variety of unrelated substances. One can only conclude that the stimulus need not be specific. It appears that any agent capable of perturbing the cell, most likely through interaction with the membrane, can set off the events leading to DNA synthesis and cell multiplication.

Multiple metabolic events following stimulation

The usual endpoint in assessing the effects of growth stimulators is either the initiation of DNA synthesis or increase in cell number. These events occur only after a delay of about 4 hours. There are, however, many events which occur very shortly after the application of stimulatory materials. A partial list of such events in the pre-replicative period is shown in Table 2.

TABLE 2a

Metabolic responses to growth stimulants

Early increase	Leakage of Ca
	Depolarization
	Glucose and AIB transport
	Uridine transport and RNA synthesis
	Phosphofructokinase activity
	Lactic acid formation
Delayed increase	Continuing glucose transport and RNA synthesis
	Protein synthesis (slight)
	Enzymes for synthesis of deoxynucleotides and DNA
	DNA synthesis
	Mitotic apparatus

TABLE 2b

Increased early uptake

Glucose
  2-deoxyglucose (3-0-methyl glucose)
Uridine
Phosphate
α-Aminoisobutyric acid
Cycloleucine
Glycine, alanine

179

No change in early uptake (or slight decrease*)
   Leucine*, phenylalanine
   Thymidine

Increased late uptake
   Thymidine (only when thymidine kinase increases)

It includes, in the case of chick embryo cells, increased
rates of transport of glucose and its analogs (18), the
amino acid analog α-amino isobutyric acid (19) (but not
leucine, strangely enough), and uridine (20). It also
includes the activation of phosphofructokinase (21),
increased production of lactic acid (21), and increased
RNA synthesis (20). The efflux of calcium is enhanced
(22). Indeed, the problem is not so much to find parameters which change, as it is to find those which do not
change--or decrease. Thus, the uptake of leucine into
acid soluble pools is unchanged or slightly decreased, and
its incorporation into protein only slightly increased.
The concentration of ATP is usually slightly decreased (23).

These are events which have been described for chick
embryo cells. The list could be expanded if other systems
were to be included. The point of all this is that the
entire state of the cell changes as a consequence of the
growth stimulating event. This event is not a simple
trigger reaction. The stimulus cannot be applied for a
short period and then removed without blocking the initiation of DNA synthesis. This was already partly apparent
in experiments in which serum addition and removal were
used to influence growth rate (24). In such experiments,
however, it is not possible to remove serum macromolecules
from the cells by simple washing because they stick firmly
to the cells, and equilibrate slowly with the medium.

This difficulty can be overcome by using pH to vary
the growth rate of cells. When this is done, it is found
that the initiation of DNA synthesis can be blocked by lowering pH at any time up to no more than a few minutes before DNA synthesis begins in cells (23). The blockage is
reversible--the upward curve for DNA synthesis resumes
where it left off if the pH is lowered for about two hours.
If lowered for five hours there is a delay of about an hour
before DNA increase resumes, and if the pH lowering is for

16 hours, the delay is about 4 hours.

Any theory of the regulation of DNA synthesis has to take these facts into account. For example, any substance whose concentration changed only transiently would not be a suitable candidate as a growth regulator, since it would presumably have triggered its train of events within that transient period (unless one of the products in the chain were unstable). The cyclic nucleotides fall into this category. One is led to the conclusion that the cell is gradually building up its biosynthetic apparatus during the pre-replicative period. At some point this buildup leads to the synthesis of enzymes specifically associated with DNA synthesis. It should be kept in mind, however, that the program of the cells is not simply to replicate DNA but to replicate the cell with all its varied components. Therefore, the changes in metabolic rates of diverse processes should not be surprising.

Substrates and processes required for the initiation of DNA synthesis

Media used for tissue culture growth are highly complex, and have been worked out in a diversity of ways. We use medium 199, which was originally developed for chick embryo cells using fairly crude methods of assay. It has many more constituents than does Eagle's medium, for example, but we find it gives more consistent and reliable results. We also add tryptose phosphate broth and serum. Of the low molecular weight components, including vitamins, purines and pyrimidines, we find that the only constituents regularly required in short term experiments for the initiation of DNA synthesis are the essential amino acids. The need for glucose in the medium is variable. Sometimes it can be dispensed with entirely and other times its concentration can be reduced 5 or 10-fold without inhibiting the initiation of DNA synthesis. The variability is probably associated with the variable content of glycogen in cells.

The major point to come out of nutritional studies, however, is that the rate of growth of cells cannot be controlled by varying the concentration of any component of the medium within limits defined by differences in the rate of uptake under different states of growth. For example, the maximum increase we detect in amino acid uptake by "turning-on" cells is a 5-fold increase in uptake of α-amino isobutyric acid. We cannot "turn-on" quiescent cells, however, by increasing the amino acid concentration of the medium, nor can we "turn-off" rapidly growing cells by decreasing the concentration of amino acids 5-fold (6, 7). Of course, we can kill the cells by depriving them of amino acids. So, while amino acids are essential for growth, their rate of uptake cannot be a major regulator of growth. The same argument can be made for glucose. Theories for growth regulation which invoke the rate of uptake of nutrients (25) are invalidated by these considerations.

The question then arises, what metabolic processes are required for the initiation of DNA synthesis? This can be examined by using metabolic inhibitors of different processes to observe effects on DNA synthesis (Table 3).

TABLE 3

Pathways required for initiation of DNA synthesis

Energy metabolism (oxidative phosphorylation)?
Ribosomal RNA synthesis
Protein synthesis

Not required
Glycolysis

Unknown
Lipid synthesis
Messenger RNA synthesis

The rate of glycolysis increases greatly after "turning-on" cells (7,21). Blocking glycolysis with NaF, iodo-acetic acid, or 2-deoxy-D-glucose, prevents the initiation of DNA synthesis (7). Unfortunately, none of these inhibitors can be considered specific for glycolysis. The first two interfere with protein and RNA synthesis (26,27), and 2-deoxy-D-glucose interferes with the formation of ATP (28). Furthermore, glycolysis can be markedly reduced by lowering the external concentration of glucose without affecting the initiation of DNA synthesis (23). We conclude therefore that the rate of glycolysis does not control the initiation of DNA synthesis.

There is indirect evidence suggesting that oxidative

phosphorylation is required for initiation of DNA synthesis. The evidence is the inhibition by 2,4-dinitrophenol of the "turn-on" of DNA synthesis. This evidence suffers from the same flaws as that obtained with inhibitors of glycolysis. It seems almost trivial, however, to anticipate that the major energy source of the cell would be required for cell replication.

The initiation of DNA synthesis is exquisitely sensitive to very low concentrations of actinomycin D (10). Concentrations so low, i.e., 0.003 µg/ml, which reputedly inhibit only ribosomal RNA synthesis, and even that only partially, have a much larger effect on the initiation of DNA synthesis. Since the effects on RNA synthesis are immediate and those on DNA synthesis are delayed, it is plausible that RNA synthesis is required to initiate DNA synthesis. But why, ribosomal RNA synthesis should be required is puzzling, and I have heard no convincing explanation.

Inhibition of protein synthesis also blocks the initiation of DNA synthesis. This is not surprising in view of the low concentration of enzymes for DNA synthesis present in quiescent cells (29). However, there are indications that protein synthesis is also needed for ongoing DNA synthesis, but this requirement does not fall into our purview of processes required to initiate DNA synthesis.

The results, therefore, indicate that RNA and protein synthesis and energy metabolism are required for the initiation of DNA synthesis. We have no information on the possible requirement of other processes such as lipid and carbohydrate synthesis for the initiation of DNA synthesis. Nor do we know whether any--or all--of these processes are involved in the regulation of cell growth.

The multiplicity of responses initiated by growth stimulators bear no apparent relationship to one another. For example, increased glucose uptake is not needed for increased RNA synthesis and vice versa (23). It appears as though the stimulatory event initiates a number of relatively independent processes. There is no indication of a linear series of events, each one dependent in its

183

turn on the preceding reaction. Only DNA synthesis itself, a very much delayed reaction, is dependent on prior events. Therefore, in speculating about the nature of the stimulatory signal we must look for an event which is capable of affecting a broad range of unrelated processes.

Simulation of events of the "turn-on" in cell-free extracts

Understanding the nature of the "turn-on" signal would be advanced if the stimulation could be done in cell-free extracts. Such events as increased transport would be difficult, if not impossible to reproduce in the absence of the intact cell. However, the activation of enzymes in metabolic sequences is subject to in vitro analysis. One such enzyme is phosphofructokinase, a key regulatory enzyme of glycolysis. In several systems, it has been found that the response of the enzyme in the intact cell to pH adjustments in the medium can be duplicated with the isolated enzyme (30). We have found similar results in the case of chick embryo cells (7,21). Phosphofructokinase is activated by small changes of pH when within, or isolated from (31) cells. The enzyme is also activated when cells are stimulated by serum, although serum does not affect the activity of the isolated enzyme.

Thus far, this is the only reaction of those occurring in vivo which has been simulated in vitro. The fact that serum produces the same changes as pH in the intact cell suggests that serum may produce its effect by raising the pH of the cell. Since the entire ensemble of reactions elicited in cells by serum is reproduced by altering pH, it would be important to establish how many of them can be reproduced in cell-free material. One way to do this is to determine, by measuring pools of intermediates, which specific enzymes are activated (or inhibited) in the intact cell within a short time after applying the "turn-on" stimulus. The sensitivity of the enzymes to pH (or any other postulated growth-mediating alteration in the cell) in cell-free extracts could then be tested.

Cyclic nucleotides

Interest in cyclic nucleotides as mediators of growth has reached a high level in the past few years (see review, 32). Much of this interest arises from the evidence that, (a) some transformed cells have a lower concentration of cyclic AMP than do normal cells. The concentration of cyclic AMP falls shortly after growth stimulation. (b) Dibutyryl cyclic AMP inhibits the growth of some cells. (c) The concentration of cyclic AMP is lower in some tumor cells than in their normal counterparts. (d) Dibutyryl cyclic AMP alters the appearance of some tumor cells to a more normal appearance.

Opposed to a central role for cyclic AMP are the following observations: In some well studied systems cyclic AMP is not inhibitory to growth. Indeed, it has been reported to stimulate growth (33). The fact that its concentration may change after stimulation is meaningless when taken by itself, since the rates of a wide diversity of reactions are changed. In several cases where the biology of the inhibitory effect of dibutyryl cyclic AMP has been studied it has been found to increase the fraction of cells in the G2 period (34). Since cells in density-inhibited cultures are chiefly in the G1 period, there is no basis for concluding that dibutyryl cyclic AMP simulates the effects of physiological inhibitors of growth.

More recently, cyclic GMP has come into prominence as a putative positive mediator of growth. The evidence here is much skimpier than in the case of cyclic AMP. This is partly due to the difficulty in measuring the low concentrations of cyclic GMP present in cells. The evidence consists of showing in a few cases that the concentration of cyclic GMP increases with growth rate (35). This can no more be considered as support for a regulatory role for cyclic GMP, than can the increase in fructose-1,6-diphosphate or of lactic acid be used to invoke their regulatory role.

Some of the thinking about the involvement of cyclic nucleotides in growth regulation seems to involve a misperception of the commonplace that differentiation and multiplication are mutually exclusive. Whatever relevance this slogan has is restricted to the period of embryological development. In the adult, the signals which call forth increased differentiated function also call forth multiplication (36). This can be seen during anoxia through accelerated multiplication of erythropoietic tissue. It is also seen in the trophic responses

185

of endocrine organs to pituitary hormones. Based on the
false dichotomy, it has been assumed that since increased
cyclic AMP is supposedly involved in stimulating differentiated function, decreased cyclic AMP must be involved
in stimulating multiplication. Aside from the questions
now being raised about the role of cyclic AMP in differentiated function of some tissues, the "atrophic"
effects of hormones might lead one to suspect that cyclic
AMP would stimulate growth in those tissues in which it
stimulates function.

These considerations should not be taken as denial of
some significant role of cyclic nucleotides in response to
growth stimulatory signals. But that role is more likely
to be just one of a panoply of responses than it is to be
the magic trigger substance. The cyclic nucleotides are
but one class of compounds out of many which have been
implicated at one time or another as being the control
substance. These incriminations are based on precon-
ceived notions, or finding a change in concentration in
different growth states. All the inferences suffer from
the same debility--they fail to meet the requirements for
rules of evidence exemplified in Koch's postulates, or to
make sense in a broad biological perspective.

Is there a singular regulatory mechanism?

Having disposed of many favorite mechanisms of growth
regulation, is there any substitute to nourish the hunger
of those who quest for an answer? If there was one available that was impervious to skeptical questioning, we would
all be aware of it by now. I have no such panacea to offer,
but I do suggest that the role of pH be closely scrutin-
ized. We have already shown that it can simulate all the
known growth regulatory effects of serum, population density and malignancy. We have also shown that it can reproduce at least one of its in vivo effects in cell free
extracts. It remains to be shown whether pH differences
do actually occur in cells in different growth states.
But, since intracellular pH is undoubtedly compartmental-
ized, its control complex and its measurement difficult,
it is unlikely that this problem will soon be solved.

For now, we can ask whether a plausible mechanism for
pH control can be invoked in physiological situations.

One possibility is as follows: pH is determined by the
rate of production of acidic substances in the cell, the
rate of their diffusion from the cell, and the buffering
capacity of the cell. I shall leave out the extra complexity of a proton pump at this stage. The chief acidic
substance produced by cells in culture is lactic acid.
Its intracellular concentration must depend to some extent
on the population density and on contact of cells, since
it will probably diffuse more readily among contiguous,
ionically coupled cells than into the medium. The rate of
release into the medium will, of course, depend on the
permeability of the membrane to anions. This has itself
been shown to increase with pH (37), so there is a positive feedback effect. In addition it has been shown that
the diffusion rate of lactic acid in muscle cells is 10
times slower than it is in extracellular space (38), so
surrounding a cell with other cells would tend to increase
the intracellular concentration of lactic acid. Any treatment which would increase the permeability of cells to
anions would speed the release of the lactic acid. Perhaps
this is what the role of the various growth stimulators
is--to simply increase the leakiness of cells (see Fig. 1).

Another possibility becomes available in the intact
tissue of the organism. This is relatively impermeable to
the bicarbonate ion, but fully permeable to CO_2 (39). If
the permeability to bicarbonate were increased, the ratio
bicarbonate: CO_2 would increase, as would pH. Increased
leakiness in the organism should increase pH both by decreasing lactic acid and increasing bicarbonate. Internal
pH could then be controlled by varying membrane permeability (Fig. 1).

The possible influence of the influx of bicarbonate
into a cell previously impermeable to this ion arises from
the fact that in accepting a proton it is converted to
H_2CO_3 and then to CO_2 which is removed from the system.
The effect of this unusual property on the buffering
capacity of bicarbonate is shown in Table 4. Even though
the pKa of bicarbonate is far below physiological pH, it
is a far better buffer in a constant pCO_2 environment than
other buffers, even those with a physiological pKa. This
can be seen in the example in Table 4, where the effects
on pH of adding 5 mM lactic acid to solutions containing

187

equal concentrations of either the organic buffer, Hepes,
or $NaHCO_3$ are analyzed. Although the Hepes solution is at
its pKa of 7.3, its pH is lowered considerably more by the
lactic acid than is the bicarbonate solution.

TABLE 4

Advantage of bicarbonate buffer in "open" system

$$pH = pKa + log \frac{[salt]}{[acid]}$$

	Hepes 25 mM	$NaHCO_3$ 25 mM
pKa (37°C)	7.3	6.1
$\left(\frac{[salt]}{[acid]}\right)$ pH 7.3	$\frac{12.5 \text{ mM}}{12.5 \text{ mM}}$	$\frac{25 \text{ mM}}{1.6 \text{ mM}}$
$\left(\frac{[salt]}{[acid]}\right)$ + 5 mM acid	$\frac{12.5 - 5}{12.5 + 5} = 0.43$	$\frac{25 - 5}{1.6} = 12.5$
pH after 5 mM acid	$7.3 - 0.37 = 6.93$	$6.1 + 1.1 = 7.2$

The effect of influx of bicarbonate into cells accumulating protons as a result of metabolism would be to raise
pH. And indeed, as Poole et al. have shown, the internal
pH of ascite tumor cells is much better buffered against
external changes in pH if bicarbonate is used in the
medium, than if phosphate buffer is used (40).

In both cases we are regulating intracellular pH by
altering the permeability of the cell membrane and allowing
lactic acid or bicarbonate to flow down their concentration
gradient. This would account for the non-specificity of
the stimulatory agents. It would also account for the
changes in permeability reported for a wide range of substances. This hypothesis does not require a large number
of ad hoc specific receptors, effectors etc., but merely
makes use of pre-existing gradients and metabolic poten-
tials. It makes predictions which are testable, and are
indeed being tested.

It remains to consider what this means for the study

of membranes and malignancy. This meeting attests to the widespread interest in both. The apposition of the two is based on the altered surface properties of cancer cells including adhesiveness to other cells, and permeability changes. It should be clear, however, that changes in membrane properties need not come about from changes in membrane constituents. Membrane function is highly responsive to the milieu of the membranes. By changing cellular metabolism, or altering the production of membrane effectors from other tissues, it would be possible to alter membrane function without changing membrane composition. This possibility needs recognition by those engaged in studying membranes from cancer cells.

Intracellular pH control
by regulation of membrane permeability

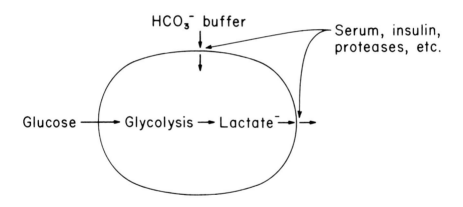

Fig. 1

REFERENCES

(1)   R. McMinn, Tissue Repair (Academic Press, New York, 1969).
(2)   H. Rubin, Cancer Res. 21 (1961) 1244.
(3)   M. Stoker and H. Rubin, Nature 215 (1967) 171.
(4)   R. Dulbecco, Nature 227 (1970) 802.
(5)   A. Rein and H. Rubin, Exp. Cell Res. 49 (1968) 666.
(6)   H. Rubin, in: Growth Control in Cell Cultures, eds. G. Wolstenholme and J. Knight (Churchill, and Livingstone, Edinburgh, 1971).
(7)   H. Rubin and D. Fodge, in: Cold Spring Harbor Symp. on Control of Proliferation in Animal Cells, eds. B. Clarkson and R. Baserga (Cold Spring Harbor, New York) in the press.
(8)   D. Fodge and H. Rubin, unpublished.
(9)   H. Rubin, Proc. Nat. Acad. Sci. 69 (1972) 712.
(10) H. Rubin and T. Koide, J. Cell Biol. 56 (1973) 777.
(11) H. Rubin, J. Cell Biol. 51 (1971) 686.
(12) H. Rubin, J. Cell Physiol. 82 (1973) 231.
(13) S. Adler, J. Clin. Invest. 51 (1972) 256.
(14) H. Rubin and T. Koide, J. Cell Physiol. 81 (1973) 387.
(15) B. Sefton and H. Rubin, Nature 227 (1970) 170.
(16) J. Vasiliev, M. Gelfand, I. Guelstein and E. Fetisova, J. Cell Physiol. 75 (1970) 305.
(17) W. Shearer, G. Philpott and C. Parker, Science 182 (1973) 1357.
(18) B. Sefton and H. Rubin, Proc. Nat. Acad. Sci. 68 (1971) 3154.
(19) D. Foster and A. Pardee, J. Biol. Chem. 244 (1969) 2675.
(20) M. Weber and H. Rubin, J. Cell Physiol. 77 (1971) 157.
(21) D. Fodge and H. Rubin, Nature New Biol. 246 (1973) 181.
(22) M. Bissell and H. Rubin, J. Cell Biol. 55 (1972) 20a.
(23) H. Rubin, unpublished.
(24) H. Temin, J. Cell Physiol. 78 (1971) 161.
(25) R. Holley, Proc. Nat. Acad. Sci. 69 (1972) 2840.
(26) H. Freudenberg and J. Mager, Biochim. Biophys. Acta 232 (1970) 537.
(27) L. Panchenko et al., Biochem. Biophys. Acta 299 (1973) 103.
(28) K. Letnansky, Biochem. Biophys. Acta 87 (1964) 1.
(29) B. Nordenskjold, L. Skoog, N. Brown and P. Reichard, J. Biol. Chem. 245 (1970) 5360.

(30) G. Wilhelm, J. Schulz and E. Hofmann, FEBS Letters 17 (1971) 158.

(31) B. Trivedi and W. Danforth, J. Biol. Chem. 241 (1966) 4110.

(32) C. Abell and T. Monahan, J. Cell Biol. 59 (1973) 549.

(33) T. Hovi and A. Vaheri, Nature New Biol. 245 (1973) 175.

(34) L. Smets, Nature New Biol. 239 (1972) 123.

(35) J. Hadden, E. Hadden, M. Haddox and N. Goldberg, Proc. Nat. Acad. Sci. 69 (1972) 3024.

(36) R. Goss, Adaptive Growth (Academic Press, New York 1964).

(37) J. Woodbury and P. Miles, J. Gen. Physiol. 62 (1973) 324.

(38) A. Hill, Proc. Roy. Soc., London (B) 104 (1929) 39.

(39) W. Wallace and A. Hastings, J. Biol. Chem. 144 (1942) 637.

(40) D. Poole, T. Butler and W. Waddell, J. Nat. Cancer Inst. 32 (1964) 939.

This investigation was supported by Public Health Service Research Grant CA 05619 from the National Cancer Institute.

DISCUSSION

W. R. Loewenstein, University of Miami: I'd like to ask Harry whether he has made any internal measurements of pH under these conditions.

H. Rubin, University of California: We have tried to measure internal pH using DMO. This does not work under our conditions of monolayer growth because there is about ten times larger volume of extracellular fluid than intracellular fluid, even after the medium has been drained. Since the DMO is readily removed from cells by washing, we must use unwashed cultures, and the presence of such a large excess of extracellular fluid makes the measurements of uptake meaningless.

W. R. Loewenstein: But microelectrodes, you haven't used?

H. Rubin: Microelectrodes have been used for measuring pH in very large muscle cells (Caldwell; Carter) and the measurements have given rise to considerable controversy of interpretation. I am afraid that the penetration of cells as small as ours by pH-sensitive microelectrodes would be much more difficult to interpret.

W.R. Loewenstein: Wouldn't one expect, on the basis of your hypothesis, that the cells be in synchrony throughout the population in all these respects, when the cells are interconnected by permeable junctions?

H. Rubin: Yes, that might cause us problems, but there would be similar problems no matter what our model of growth control was as long as we were invoking changes in concentration of small molecules, or ions, as a controlling element. It becomes a question of whether all cells are equivalent in ionically coupled populations. The fact that there is a considerable range of membrane

potential values indicates that considerable variation in
ion concentration is possible in such a cell population.
(O'Lague and Rubin in "Growth Control in Cell Culture".
Ciba Foundn. Symp. edited by Wolstenholme and Knight
(1971), p. 257. Churchill Livingstone, Edinburgh).

J. Hochstadt, Worcester Foundation for Experimental
Biology: I'm very glad that you have given us the caveat
of trying to distinguish between membrane-specific changes
and subsequent metabolic effects. Having a great respect
for this idea, about a year and a half ago, after having
studied bacterial membrane transport mechanisms for five
years, I went back to a technique I had used while I was
a fellow in Don Wallach's laboratory eight years ago, and
began to make membrane vesicles from established mammalian
cell lines. These preprations have included both isolated
plasma membrane vesicles separated from endoplasmic reticulum, as well as of total endoplasmic and surface membrane vesicles. I'd like to make a few comments about
the work of Dr. Dennis Quinlan in my laboratory has been
doing with Balb/c 3T3 cells. First of all, before he
started he was aware of the results of Ceccarini and
Eagle and has controlled the pH throughout his experiments.
He has isolated membrane vesicles from both subconfluent
log phase cells of Balb/c 3T3 and also the confluent or
stationary cells of the same 3T3 and he has been able
to repeat in isolated membrane vesicles the uridine results
that Cunningham and Pardee obtained for whole cells. He
has also found that adenosine uptake did not differ when
the vesicles prepared from growing cells were compared to
vesicles prepared from contact inhibited cultures. This
too is consistent with the results of Cunningham and
Pardee. Thus we can state that at least for uridine and
adenosine transport, growth dependent variations observed
in whole cells can be attributed to differences in uptake
demonstrable in isolated plasma membrane vesicles and thus
would represent changes in the membrane itself.

A. H. Romano, University of Connecticut: First of
all, I'm glad to hear that you ascribe at least a part
of the apparent increase in deoxyglucose uptake to the
dragging effect of glycolysis. My specific question,
however, deals with the rapid increase in activity of

phosphofructokinase. Do you mean here the specific activity as measured by in vitro activity, or do you mean
the in vivo measurement of the activity?

H. Rubin: It is an in vivo measurement based on
analysis of concentrations of glycolytic intermediates by
the cross over technique, and by changes in mass action
ratios.

A. H. Romano: So essentially what you're talking
about is an allosteric regulation.

H. Rubin: Correct.

A. H. Romano: Thank you.

J. Roth, Biocenter, Switzerland: I'd like to ask
two questions about the amino acid transport experiments.
The first question is: Considering the fact that even
though you didn't observe very quick initiation of DNA
synthesis in response to serum stimulations, you did
observe a very quick increase of deoxyglucose transport
which you said was entered in a period of less than one
minute. Considering the fact that most, if not all, of
the amino acid transport experiments in the literature have
utilized two conditions, the starvation of amino acids
and the absence of serum, is it really valid to measure
amino acid transport under these conditions considering
the fact that within that period of time you could already
be looking at inhibition of the transport?

H. Rubin: Our experiments on amino acid transport
have been done in our complete growth medium, so we could
be certain we were looking at uptake under the conditions
of the experiment.

J. Roth: Leucine transport with serum?

H. Rubin: Yes. In this context I should cite the
paper of Wiebel and Baserga (J. Cell Physio. 74, 191
[1969]) who also measured amino acid uptake without
starving for amino acids, and found a decreased rate of
uptake after serum stimulation.

J. *Roth*: One other point on the transport media that I'd like to ask about is bicarbonate because in many cases people have used phosphate buffered saline in which they do their transport studies, and don't normally use bicarbonate, which you pointed out has great importance in the control of pH.

H. *Rubin*: We have used Good's organic buffers as well as bicarbonate, and get the same results.

M. *Lubin, Dartmouth Medical School*: You noted that cyclic AMP had no effect as a growth inhibitor. Many other laboratories, however, have noted an antagonism between serum and dibutyryl cyclic AMP, I wonder, therefore, if you looked at a variety of serum concentrations?

H. *Rubin*: Dibutyryl cyclic AMP has no effect on the initiation of DNA synthesis in chick cells even at very low external serum concentrations, where the cells are stimulated by raising pH. This despite the use of millimolar concentrations of the "inhibitor".

M. *Lubin*: But when serum was limiting, did you....

H. *Rubin*: Strangely enough, Hovi and Vaheri have found that cyclic AMP has a slight stimulatory effect on the growth of chick embryo cells (Nature New Biol. 245, 175 [1973]).

M.J. *Weber, University of Illinois*: I'd like to comment on that. Vaheri has found that dibutyryl cyclic AMP actually stimulates the growth of chick cells, in the absence of theophylline, and we've confirmed that result.

H. *Rubin*: Well, it doesn't stimulate ours, but it certainly doesn't inhibit it.

M.J. *Weber*: Well, using the transformed cells, it actually stimulated.

M. *Morrison, St. Jude Children's Research Hospital*: The question of changes in the membrane as a function of pH has come up repeatedly in this meeting. We have actually studied plasma membrane changes as a function of pH.

195

With our favorite membrane probe, lactoperoxidase macromolecular probe system, and our favorite model membrane
system, the red cell plasma membrane. We studied changes
in the pH range from 6 to 8.5. There is a marked alteration in the accessibility of membrane components on the
external surface of the membrane as a function of pH.
The major glycoprotein becomes much less accessible to the
lactoperoxidase probe at low pH values, while a low molecular weight component which is not accessible to the
lactoperoxidase probe at high pH values becomes very
accessible, so in this system at least, marked changes
in external proteins of plasma membrane do take place.
One other point has come up in both your discussion, Dr.
Rubin and Dr. Eagle's discussion was the effect of prolonged pH changes. These changes that I've just discussed
are reversible over short time periods, but at longer
periods are not reversible.

   H. Rubin: Growth in our cells can be stimulated even
after several days at as low a pH as 6.5, by raising pH.
Of course, our cells are metabolically considerably more
versatile than are red blood cells.

   H. Eagle, Albert Einstein College of Medicine: Dr.
Morrison, when you say that the membrane changes resulting from prolonged exposure to e.g., low pH are non-
reversible, how long have these cells been followed?

   M. Morrison: Although we haven't studied it in great
detail, I'm talking about days.

REGULATION OF CYCLIC NUCLEOTIDE LEVELS BY PHOSPHODIESTERASE

MARK W. BITENSKY, NAOMASA MIKI, JAMES J. KEIRNS
and FRED R. MARCUS
Department of Pathology
Yale University School of Medicine

ABSTRACT: The role of cyclic nucleotides in determining cell surface characteristics and mitotic behavior has been intensively studied. However the capacity of phosphodiesterase to regulate intracellular cyclic nucleotide concentrations is often neglected. We describe a single phosphodiesterase in vertebrate photoreceptors which is activated by light and ATP and which can markedly alter the ratio of cyclic AMP and cyclic GMP in the same cells.

INTRODUCTION

This report emphasizes the importance and efficacy of the enzyme phosphodiesterase as a regulator of the intracellular levels of cAMP* and cGMP*. There has been great interest in the effects of cyclic nucleotides on the rates of cell division and on cell surface characteristics in normal and cancer cells (1, 2, 3).

*Abbreviations: cAMP - adenosine 3',5' cyclic monophosphate, cGMP - guanosine 3',5' cyclic monophosphate.

197

We believe that in the evaluation of cyclic
nucleotide function in a variety of cell types,
the role of cyclic nucleotide phosphodiesterase
has often been neglected. We therefore offer a
caveat which is intrinsic in our findings to
emphasize the importance of fully evaluating
phosphodiesterase activities in describing a
cyclic nucleotide regulatory paradigm in normal,
transformed or neoplastic cells.

In 1970 we initiated studies on the role of
cyclic nucleotides in the regulation of photoreceptor function (4). Our data seemed
compatible with the idea that cyclic nucleotides
could regulate the sensitivity of the photoreceptor much in analogy to the regulation of the
sensitivity of cerebellar Purkinje cells by
cyclic nucleotides (5). The evidence indicated
that in suspensions of outer segment disc
membranes light could diminish the synthesis of
cAMP from radioactive ATP, and that light did
not influence the activity of phosphodiesterase
in these preparations. We therefore concluded
that the locus of regulation was adenyl cyclase
and originally suggested that as a promising
mechanism for the explanation of light dark
adaptation in vertebrate photoreceptors (4,6,7).

These ideas have persisted and have been
strengthened by much additional evidence (8,9,
10,11). We are now confident indeed that cyclic
nucleotides fluctuate as a function of
illumination in a manner which could influence
the sensitivity of the outer segments of many
different vertebrate photoreceptors (11).
However we have been compelled by recent findings
(9,10,11) to alter the intepretation of our
earlier studies specifically in regard to the
locus of light regulation. We now conclude
that the actual regulator of cyclic nucleotide
concentrations in the outer segment of the
photoreceptor is phosphodiesterase (10).

The reason that we were mislead in our initial studies of the photoreceptor cyclic nucleotide system related to the unusual circumstance that the activation of photo-receptor phosphodiesterase by light is uniquely dependent on the presence of ATP or another nucleoside triphosphate (9). Thus when one measures phosphodiesterase activity in this system, using outer segment disc membranes in the absence of ATP, there is no measurable effect of light on phosphodiesterase. The omission of ATP from a reaction mix for the assay of phosphodiesterase is customary since ATP is not only unnecessary for the measurement of phosphodiesterase but at concentrations above 2mM can actually act as a competitive inhibitor. These exceptional circumstances which are necessary for the light activation of photoreceptor phosphodiesterase prevented an assignment of the true locus of light regulation of photoreceptor cyclic nucleotide levels for some time, even though other laboratories had joined in the study of cyclic nucleotide metabolism in retinal tissues (12,13,14,15).

There are other examples where phosphodiesterase regulation can markedly alter the levels of cyclic nucleotides in various tissues. Especially important in this regard is Kakiuchi's finding that calcium can regulate the activity of neuronal phosphodiesterase in a dramatic fashion (16). Kakiuchi has shown that, in the presence of a purified protein regulator, calcium can activate neuronal phosphodiesterase as much as 10 fold (17). There have also been reports that insulin can influence the activity of phosphodiesterase in liver and fat (18,19). In addition there is evidence that cGMP may enhance the hydrolysis of cAMP (20). Further, the ambient levels of cyclic nucleotides in a cell can regulate the total numbers of phosphodiesterase enzymes synthesized (21). This effect appears to depend on the participa-tion of a cAMP dependent protein kinase (22).

This report will describe in detail the unique events of the light activation of the photoreceptor phosphodiesterase. This regulation of phosphodiesterase appears especially attractive as a modulator in excitable tissue and involves the participation of light, rhodopsin, a nucleoside triphosphate, the photoreceptor phosphodiesterase (inactive) and a membrane bound phosphodiesterase activator. We also compare the properties of this photoreceptor phosphodiesterase to the phosphodiesterases of other tissues. Although photoreceptor membranes contain phosphodiesterase activities which can hydrolyze both cAMP and cGMP, both these activities probably reside in a single protein which has a marked preference for cGMP. We also show how the regulation of this single protein can markedly alter the ratio of cGMP to cAMP and finally we estimate the quantitative relationships among all of the adenine and guanine cyclic nucleotide related enzymes in the photoreceptor.

MATERIALS AND METHODS

All dark manipulations were accomplished using near infrared light and infrared image converters in the complete absence of visible light (11). Large Rana catesbiana were dark adapted for 12 hours and decapitated. Photoreceptor outer segment membranes were prepared from the retinas by floatation on 47% sucrose as previously described (9). Adenyl and guanyl cyclases and phosphodiesterases were measured using tritiated substrates. Products were isolated using thin layer chromatography as previously described (9,23). Thin layer isolates were combusted in an Oxymat (Intertechnique) prior to scintillation counting (23). The reaction mixture for cyclase included tritiated ATP or GTP as substrate and 0.5mM isobutylmethylxanthine as a phosphodiesterase inhibitor and otherwise was as previously described (9). The phosphodiesterase reaction

mixture included tritiated cAMP or cGMP   (5mM)
and 1mM ATP.   Cyclase assays were incubated at
30° for 5 minutes and phosphodiesterase assays
were incubated at 30° for 1 minute.   Reactions
were terminated by boiling for 2 minutes.
Protein kinase was assayed with $[\gamma-^{32}P]ATP$ by
the method of Kuo and Greengard (27).   Opsin
kinase was assayed in illuminated membranes with
no added histone.   Histone kinase was measured
in the dark with unilluminated membranes and
1mg/ml. calf thymus histone (Sigma type II-A).

RESULTS

Sensitivity of the system to light: The
sensitivity of the photoreceptor phosphodiesterase to illumination is shown in Fig. 1.
In this experiment the totally bleached and
unbleached (fully dark adapted and never
illuminated) photoreceptor membranes are mixed
in varying proportions in order to evaluate
the effects of different quantities of
illumination on the activation sequence.   It is
seen that even with as little as a 2% admixture
of bleached photoreceptor membranes the
phosphodiesterase is maximally activated.
Similar results were obtained by exposing the
fully dark adapted photoreceptor disc membrane
vesicles to light for various time periods and
estimating the extent of bleaching spectropho-
metrically.   The latter design differed from
the mixing experiment in that the bleached
rhodopsins were uniformally distributed through
the disc membranes while in the mixing
experiment, the majority of the disc membranes
were entirely in the unilluminated state and a
small fraction were entirely in the illuminated
state.   Both designs however gave very
comparable results and illustrated the marked
sensitivity of the photoreceptor systems to
small quantities of illumination, i.e. to
minute quantities of bleached rhodopsin
irrespective of the pattern of distribution of
the rhodopsin in the disc membranes.

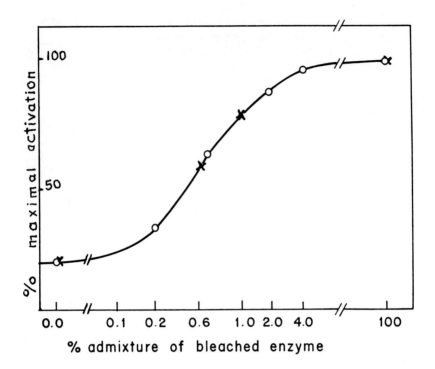

Fig. 1. Dependence of photoreceptor phosphodiesterase activity on light. Photoreceptor membranes were isolated in the dark. Part were fully bleached in room light and part held in the dark. Mixtures of illuminated and unilluminated membranes were prepared (with the percentage of bleached material indicated on the abscissa above) and assayed for cAMP (o) or cGMP (x) phosphodiesterase activities. The activities are expressed as percent of the maximal (100% bleached) activity for the given substrate.

TABLE 1

Light-dependent and ATP-dependent steps of
Phosphodiesterase Activation

	Phosphodiesterase Activity
No ATP present	0.8 ± 0.1
0.8mM ATP present during bleaching but diluted to 0.006mM before assay	0.8 ± 0.1
0.8mM ATP present only during assay	4.2 ± 0.2
0.8mM ATP present during both bleaching and assay	4.2 ± 0.2

Phosphodiesterase activity (μmoles cAMP destroyed/min/mg protein) is measured in a mixture of 2% illuminated-98% unilluminated photoreceptor membranes. The specific activity of illuminated material was 4.3 ± 0.2 and for the unilluminated material 0.8 ± 0.1.

Resolution of the excitation sequence into a minimum of two steps: During the actual illumination of the disc membranes it is not necessary to have a nucleoside triphosphate present. A nucleoside triphosphate must be added prior to assay, however, since in its absence the phosphodiesterase is not activated. On the other hand if the nucleoside triphosphate is present during illumination, but is removed by washing or dilution prior to mixing the illuminated and unilluminated membranes, no activation is observed. These facts are summarized in Table 1.

Figure 2 illustrates the concentration requirements for nucleoside triphosphates in the light activation of photoreceptor phosphodiesterase. At higher concentrations, ATP inhibits the phosphodiesterase activity. On the other hand, CTP can replace ATP in the activation sequence but does not inhibit phosphodiesterase at higher concentrations. This probably reflects the greater resemblance of ATP to the purine substrates of phosphodiesterase.

Structure activity relationships of nucleoside triphosphates and analogues: Table 2 contains a list of various phosphate compounds which have been evaluated for their ability to participate in the activation sequence. It will be noted that the requirements thus far established include either a purine or pyrimidine base, and a ribose (or deoxyribose) triphosphate. Phosphate compounds which depart from this general plan (except for adenosine tetraphosphate and alpha-beta, methylene ATP) are ineffective. Beta-gamma, methylene ATP is totally without effect and adenylylimidodiphosphate, a compound where nitrogen replaces oxygen between the beta and gamma phosphates produces a slight effect. Inorganic polyphosphates, purine nucleoside mono- and diphosphates and other high energy compounds (e.g. creatine phosphate, phosphoenol pyruvate) are without effect.

Characteristics of the activator: The mixing design permits manipulations of the small fraction of illuminated membranes without influencing the bulk of the phosphodiesterase in the unilluminated membrane fraction. Using this approach we found that the activator was stable to trypsin, phospholipase C, and dialysis, but was compromised by heating (5 minutes at 90°), and by Triton X-100. Heating at 60° for 20 minutes selectively damages phosphodiesterase and not the activator.

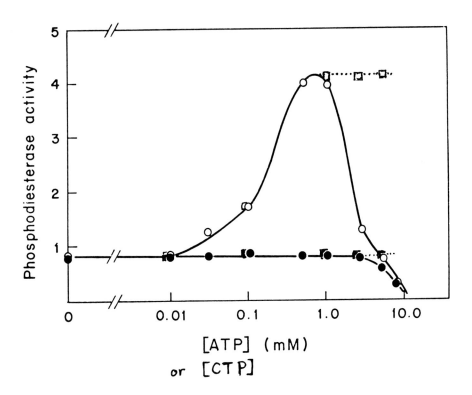

Fig. 2. Dependence of photoreceptor phosphodiesterase activity on nucleoside triphosphate concentration. cAMP phosphodiesterase activity was assayed with the indicated concentration of ATP and illuminated (o) or unilluminated (●) photoreceptor membranes. Assays were also performed with the indicated concentration of CTP and illuminated (□) or unilluminated (■) photoreceptor membranes. Similar data were obtained for cGMP phosphodiesterase activity (same half maximal value for ATP or CTP)

TABLE 2

Requirement for nucleoside triphosphates

(1mM)	Phosphodiesterase Activity	
	Dark	Light
None	0.5	0.5
ATP, deoxy ATP CTP, deoxy CTP GTP, deoxy GTP ITP Adenosine tetraphosphate	0.5	4.1
UTP TTP	0.5 0.5	3.6 3.0
Adenylyl imidodiphosphate β-γ methylene ATP α-β methylene ATP	0.5 0.5 0.5	0.8 0.5 1.4
Phosphoenol pyruvate Phosphoribosyl pyrophosphate (PRPP) Creatine phosphate Thiamine triphosphate* AMP ADP	0.5	0.5
Pyrophosphate (Na) Tripolyphosphate (Na)	0.5	0.5

The methylene ATP compounds were purchased from PL Biochemicals, Adenylyl imidodiphosphate from ICN Chemicals and the others from Sigma Chemical Company.

* a gift from Dr. J.R. Cooper, Yale School of Medicine.

TABLE 3

Susceptibility of the phosphodiesterase
stimulator or of the phosphodiesterase
to various treatments

Treatment	Phosphodiesterase Activity	
	2% Light treated	98% Dark treated
None	3.1	3.1
Trypsin digestion	3.3	0.01
Phospholipase C digestion	3.0	3.1
Heating (60°, 20 min.)	3.0	0.01
Heating (90°, 10 min.)	0.7	0.01
Dialysis against 0.5mM EGTA	3.0	3.0
0.5% Triton X-100	0.7	0.7

Phosphodiesterase activity (μmoles cAMP destroy-
ed/min/mg protein) is measured in a mixture of
2% illuminated - 98% unilluminated photoreceptor
membranes. The specific activity of unilluminated membranes is 0.7 and of illuminated
membranes 3.2.

These characteristics of the phosphodiesterase
activator are summarized in Table 3. The
activator sediments with the rhodopsin fraction
in continuous sucrose gradients (Table 4).

TABLE 4

The activation of photoreceptor phosphodiesterase by bleached disc membrane fragments fractionated on a continuous sucrose gradient: Unilluminated photoreceptor disc membranes (suspended in 10mM Tris buffer, pH 7.5) were heated at 60° for 20 minutes causing complete loss of phosphodiesterase activity, but no loss of activator function. This material was layered on a continuous sucrose gradient (12% to 40%) and centrifuged for 1 hour at 100,000xg. Then the tube was exposed to light and four fractions taken as shown below. Fraction 1 is the buffer in which the membranes were originally suspended. Fraction 3 is the red zone. The activator fractions were assayed by mixing (5%) with unbleached intact disc membranes (95%) and assayed for phosphodiesterase in the dark with 1mM ATP. This activity is given below as "activating capacity". The percent of the total rhodopsin in each fraction was estimated spectrophotometrically.

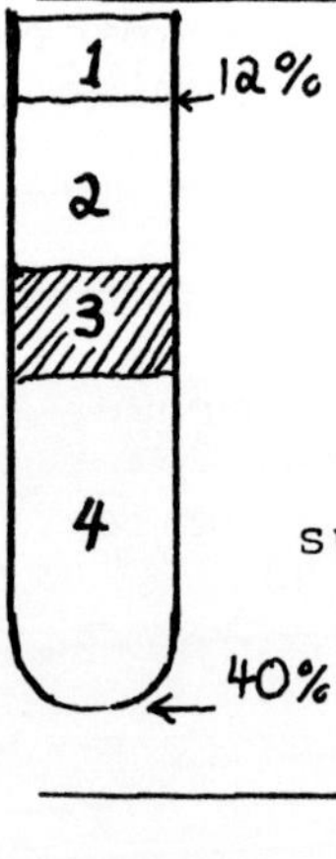

Fraction number	Activating capacity	% of total rhodopsin
1	0.60	< 1
2	0.61	< 1
3 (red)	4.2	> 95
4	0.61	< 1
suspension buffer	0.61	None

(Tube diagram on left, labeled 1, 2, 3, 4 with 12% at top and 40% at bottom)

Comparison of cGMP and cAMP phosphodiesterase activities: The photoreceptor membranes exhibit both cGMP and cAMP phosphodiesterase activities. However, at those cyclic nucleotide concentrations which prevail in the cell (less than 1μM) the relative rates of hydrolysis, cGMP/cAMP are 23 to 1. This is explained in terms of the Km's for the substrates which are 0.15mM for cGMP and 8mM for cAMP (11). These data raised the question of whether the photoreceptor membranes contained separate cGMP and cAMP phosphodiesterases or whether both activities reside in the same protein. In order to approach this question we compared a variety of stimulators and inhibitors for their effects on both the cGMP and cAMP phosphodiesterases.

Both the mixing curve which quantitatively depicts light activation (Figure 1) and the nucleoside triphosphate curve (Figure 2) have the same characteristics (half maximal effects are achieved at the same point for either cAMP or cGMP in both bleaching and ATP concentration curves) whether cAMP or cGMP are used as substrates. Imidazole which is known to activate phosphodiesterase in several different tissues (24) has no effect on either cAMP or cGMP phosphodiesterase in this system. Finally the percent inhibition found with varying amounts of such inhibitors as heat, detergent or mercurials are identical for the hydrolysis of both cyclic nucleotides (Table 5).

Another indication of the simplicity of the photoreceptor phosphodiesterase is the presence of a single Km for each substrate in contrast to both high and low Kms found for phosphodiesterases in many other tissues (25). These data suggest that a single membrane affiliated phosphodiesterase hydrolyzes both cGMP and cAMP and is activated by a single membrane affiliated regulator. The affinity characteristics of the catalytic moiety of

209

TABLE 5

Effects of various inhibitors on cAMP and
cGMP phosphodiesterase activities

Inhibitor or Treatment	Percent of control activity:	
	cAMP hydrolysis	cGMP hydrolysis
None	100%	100%
Heating (60°, 20 min)	0%	0%
(40°, 20 min)	31%	29%
p-mercuribenzoate		
(10^{-6}M)	90%	92%
(10^{-5}M)	23%	24%
(10^{-4}M)	13%	13%
Triton X-100 (0.5%)	0%	0%
(0.1%)	83%	79%
Isobutylmethylxanthine	37%	39%

cAMP and cGMP phosphodiesterase activities were
measured with illuminated photoreceptor membranes
following the given treatment or in the presence
of the given inhibitor. Control activity for
cAMP was 2μmoles/min/mg and for cGMP was 4 μmoles
/min/mg.

this enzyme suggest that in vivo cGMP is
probably the natural substrate.

Other enzymatic components in the
photoreceptor membranes: In addition to the
phosphodiesterase which is described above we
have measured both adenyl and guanyl cyclases
and both cGMP and cAMP dependent protein
kinases. The specific activities and estimated

amounts (per rod) of these enzymes are shown in
Table 6. To estimate the numbers of enzymes,
turnover numbers of 100 substrates converted/
min/enzyme were assumed as well as 1.2×10^{16}
rhodopsins/mg protein, 2×10^{6} rhodopsins/disc and
3000 discs/rod. The point to be emphasized
here are that there appears to be a slightly
greater ability to synthesize cGMP than cAMP and,
more significantly, the relative abundance of
phosphodiesterase suggests a formidable capacity
to hydrolyze cyclic nucleotides, a capacity
appropriate for the major regulatory role in the
photoreceptor. Further as a consequence of the
activation of photoreceptor phosphodiesterase
one would expect a very profound and rapid
decline of cyclic GMP concentrations and a much
smaller decline in the cyclic AMP concentration.
As a result of these events the ratio of cGMP to
cAMP would fall dramatically following the
activation of a single photoreceptor
phosphodiesterase. The rapid change in the
ratio of the 2 cyclic nucleotides which follows
upon phosphodiesterase activation is
illustrated in Figure 3.

DISCUSSION

    In the photoreceptor outer-segment membranes
there is an apparatus which can produce a marked
light and nucleoside triphosphate dependent
activation of photoreceptor phosphodiesterase.
This activation is primarily responsible for the
fluctuation of cyclic nucleotide concentrations
as a function of illumination. When precautions
are taken for the removal of phosphodiesterase
activity, the adenyl cyclase exhibits no light
sensitivity.

    The regulatory importance of cGMP
phosphodiesterase is emphasized by the fact that
the tissue has a much better facility to
hydrolyze cGMP than to produce it. The data
suggests that both cAMP and cGMP
phosphodiesterase activities reside in a single

211

TABLE 6

Specific activities and estimated numbers of enzyme
molecules in frog rod outer segments

Enzyme	V_{max} (μmole/min /mg protein)	Number of enzymes (TN = 100)		
		/rhodopsin	/disc	/rod
cAMP or cGMP phosphodiesterase (with light & ATP)	4	1×10^{-4}	200	6×10^5
Adenyl cyclase	0.00014	3×10^{-9}	0.007	21
Guanyl cyclase	0.0003	6×10^{-9}	0.015	45
Opsin kinase	20	5×10^{-4}	1000	3×10^6
Histone kinase	0.8	2×10^{-5}	40	1×10^5
Δ with 10^{-6} M cAMP	0.4	2×10^{-5}	20	5×10^4
Δ with 10^{-6} M cGMP	0.4	1×10^{-5}	20	5×10^4

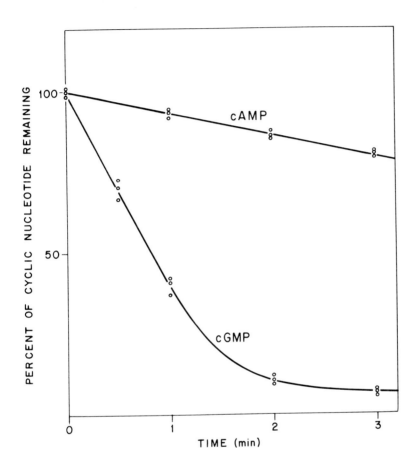

Fig. 3. Effect of abrupt activation
of photoreceptor phosphodiesterase
on cyclic nucleotide concentrations.
The concentrations of cAMP and cGMP
are assumed to be equal initially.
Within a short time however, the ratio
of cAMP to cGMP becomes rather large.

enzyme in this tissue. The unique dependence on a nucleoside triphosphate and light sets this phosphodiesterase apart from all other known phosphodiesterases.

A protein kinase probably does not participate in the activation sequence since exogenous protein kinases do not produce the activation of photoreceptor phosphodiesterases in the dark, and since activation of the phosphodiesterase by light and ATP is not prevented by 5mM adenosine which inhibits the various protein kinase activities of the photoreceptor membranes (histone kinase is 80% inhibited and opsin kinase 99% inhibited).

Since calcium has been suggested as an intermediate between photon capture and visual excitation (26), we examined the possibility that calcium mediates the activation of phosphodiesterase by light. However activation occurs in the presence of chelators of calcium and calcium itself does not mimic the effects of light in this system (11).

The source of the cyclic nucleotides which are hydrolyzed in the outer segment is not definitively known. Although we have some evidence for cyclase activity associated with the outer segment membranes (8,10) we cannot exclude the possibility that the bulk of the cyclic nucleotides are produced in the inner segment and diffuse into the outer segment (as ATP is believed to do). The diffusion would be aided by the fact that the photoreceptor has the characteristics of an electroporesis cell with the inner segment negatively charged relative to the outer segment.

We emphasize that in order to evaluate the regulation of cyclic nucleotides in any tissue one must carefully measure the phosphodiesterase under a variety of different experimental conditions and fully account for its specific activity, its susceptibility to activators and inhibitors and its relative preponderence as compared to the synthetic capacity of the cyclase in order to finally and correctly assign regulatory roles to the various enzymes of the cyclase cascade.

REFERENCES

(1) A.W. Hsie, C. Jones, T.T. Puck, Proc. Nat. Acad. Sci. USA 68 (1971) 1648.

(2) P. Furmanski, D.J. Silverman, M. Lubin, Nature 233 (1971) 413.

(3) G.S. Johnson, R.M. Friedman, I. Pastan, Proc. Nat. Acad. Sci. USA 68 (1971) 425.

(4) M.W. Bitensky, R.E. Gorman, W.H. Miller, Proc. Nat. Acad. Sci. USA 68 (1971) 561.

(5) G.R. Siggins, B.J. Hoffer, F.E. Bloom, Science 165 (1969) 1018.

(6) W.H. Miller, R.E. Gorman, M.W. Bitensky, Science 174 (1971) 295

(7) M.W. Bitensky, R.E. Gorman, W.H. Miller, Science 175 (1972) 1363.

(8) M.W. Bitensky, J.J. Keirns, R.C. Wagner, in: Biochemistry and Physiology of Visual Pigments, ed. H. Langer (Springer-Verlag, Berlin, 1973) p. 335.

(9) N. Miki, J.J. Keirns, F.R. Marcus, M.W. Bitensky, Exper. Eye Res., in press.

(10) M.W. Bitensky, N. Miki, F.R. Marcus, J.J. Keirns, Life Sci. 13 (1973) 1451.

(11) N. Miki, J.J. Keirns, F.R. Marcus, M.W. Bitensky, Proc. Nat. Acad. Sci. USA 70 (1973) in press.

(12)   D. Bounds, J. Dawes, J. Miller, in:
        Biochemistry and Physiology of Visual
        Pigments, ed. H. Langer (Springer-Verlag,
        Berlin, 1973) p. 267.

(13)   R.G. Pannbacker, Science 182 (1973) 1138.

(14)   R.E. Bensinger, R.T. Fletcher, G.T. Chader,
        Science 183 (1974) 86.

(15)   C. Goridis, N. Virmaux, P.F. Urban, P.
        Mandel, FEBS Letters 30 (1973) 163.

(16)   S. Kakiuchi, R. Yamazaki, Y. Teshima,
        Advances in Cyclic Nucleotide Research 1
        (1973) 455.

(17)   S. Kakiuchi, R. Yamazaki, Y. Teshima, K.
        Uenishi, Proc. Nat. Acad. Sci. USA 70
        (1973) 3526.

(18)   M. Vaughan, in: Insulin Action, ed. I.B.
        Fritz (Academic Press, New York, 1972)
        p. 297.

(19)   P.D.R. House, P. Poulis, M.J. Weideman,
        Eur. J. Biochem. 24 (1972) 429.

(20)   U. Klotz, K. Stock, N.S. Arch. Pharm. 274
        (1972) 54.

(21)   M. D'Armento, G.S. Johnson, I. Pastan, Proc.
        Nat. Acad. Sci. USA 69 (1972) 459.

(22)   H.R. Bourne, G.M. Tomkins, S. Dion,
        Science 181 (1973) 952.

(23)   J.J. Keirns, M.W. Bitensky, Anal. Biochem.,
        in press.

(24)   R.W. Butcher, E.W. Sutherland, J. Biol.
        Chem. 237 (1962) 1244

(25)   A.L. Pichard, J. Hanoune, J.C. Kaplan,
       Biochim. Biophys. Acta 315 (1973) 370.

(26)   S. Yoshikami and W.A. Hagins, in:
       Biochemistry and Physiology of Visual
       Pigments, ed. H. Langer (Springer-Verlag,
       Berlin, 1973) p. 245.

(27)   J.F. Kuo and P. Greengard, J. Biol. Chem.
       245 (1970) 2493.

This work was supported by USPHS grants
AM15016 and CA13444, by The American Cancer
Society grant BC-106C and by the grant from the
Jane Coffin Childs Memorial Fund for Medical
Research. J.J. Keirns is a fellow of the Jane
Coffin Childs Memorial Fund for Medical Research.

DISCUSSION

B. F. Erlanger, Columbia University: In your abstract you make some comment about the nature of the activator. I was hoping you would present additional data but you haven't said anything in your talk about it. I wonder if you have additional information.

M. W. Bitensky, Yale University: Because of the mixing design, one can functionally isolate an activator as a small fraction of illuminated membranes which when mixed with the bulk of the unilluminated membranes activates the phosphodiesterase in the unilluminated membranes. Then one can subject this small illuminated fraction to a variety of insults and then evaluate it for residual activation capacity. It appears to be completely unaffected by dialysis. It is sensitive to 0.5% Triton X-100, it is also sensitive to heating. Heating to 90° for 5 minutes completely inactivates the activator. However, the phosphodiesterase is even more sensitive to heating. If we heat the membranes for about 10 minutes at 60° we can totally inactivate phosphodiesterase and still preserve activating function of those membranes so that one can functionally separate the phosphodiesterase activity and the activation potential.

B. F. Erlanger: Just one other question. Would you be willing to speculate on what rhodopsin is doing to produce this activation? Do you have any information on this at all?

M. W. Bitensky: First of all, rhodopsin and the activator of phosphodiesterase are not yet functionally separable, that is, they sediment together. The wavelength of light most effective in bleaching rhodopsin is also most effective in activating phosphodiesterase. In addition both rhodopsin and activator exhibit sulfhydryl chemistry, that is, bleaching of rhodopsin exposes

218

sulfhydryls and activator is sensitive to agents which attack sulfhydryls (pCMB).

P. A. Srere, Veterans Administration Hospital: I'm not familiar with the volumes that are being occuppied in the cells that are being talked about, but I'd like to point out that if you have 6 million molecules of anything in an ordinary animal cell, you're talking about are overall concentration of 10^{-5} to 6×10^{-5} molar and if you have 6 million molecules of the phosphodiesterase and it has a considerable binding capacity for any one of the cyclic AMP, then it's going to have enormous effect on the free concentration of these cellular compounds.

M. W. Bitensky: Well, I would like to say two things in reply to that. The volume of a frog rod outer segment is about 300 μm^3 so the concentration of enzyme would be 10^{-9} or 10^{-8} molar. But I think that there has to be substantial uncertainty in the estimation of these numbers because they're based on an assumed turnover number of 100 molecules of substrate per minute. However, since the phosphodiesterase there we're looking at is so profoundly sensitive to light and is light regulated, I think that this influence that it would have on ambient cyclic nucleotide concentrations would be light-sensitive. I don't think the affinity for the substrate would be constant, but I would like to say that in its active form (in the light) it would bind and that in its non-active form (in the dark) it wouldn't.

P. A. Srere: While it's true that K_m does not equal K_s, it is interesting that your K_m does not vary in terms of the activation when you go from dark to light.

M. W. Bitensky: Could I reply to that question? I think you pointed out something very interesting I would be inclined to say that we are looking at some sort of basal activity before we shine light on the system, because there's phosphodiesterase without illumination. And I think that in a sense that may confuse the appearance of the kinetics. I think there may be no affinity. In other words, it would appear from the kinetics that the dark or unilluminated system has the same affinity as the illuminated system. I would suspect that the dark enzyme

has no affinity whatsoever and that the apparent affinity
that we see in the unilluminated system as basal activity,
may represent phosphodiesterase either from the inner
segment or phosphodiesterase that's been damaged in
preparation. If you're really careful about all the
conditions, you can see as much as a 30-fold activation.
I rather suspect that one could get this even lower, and
that there's virtually nothing there in the unilluminated
state.

J. Kallos, Columbia University: I would like to make
a short comment regarding use of immobilized cyclic AMP
as a probe for cell surfaces, and for examining the
biological activity of cyclic AMP by acting directly on the
membranes of cultured cells. The general questions related to the role of cyclic AMP were extensively discussed
last year, but we know very little really about what cylic
AMP does and how it acts on the cell. In order to examine
this question as to whether cyclic AMP acts always inside
of the cell or whether it acts on cell membranes we have
used immobilized cyclic AMP attached to agarose beads. We
ask simply the question whether or not this can produce
action similar to fully solubilized cyclic AMP. The
results seems to imply that not only is it logically active,
but in fact it is more active than it's soluble counterpart. Here, in the next two minutes I just want to show
you one single result examining the effect of cyclic AMP
immobilizing. For example, Shepherd has shown that cyclic
AMP in solution at very high concentrations can affect cell
growth. Okay, we have an immobilized cyclic AMP attached
by the 6 amino end to beads in the culture cell. For
example, with L and 3T3 cells transformed by polioma 10^{-4}
molar soluble cyclic AMP does not appear to have too much
effect on control of cell growth. But even 10^{-6} molar
immobilized cyclic AMP establishes control of cell growth
and also affects the transport and many of the cell
phenomena. In addition in terms of molecular events, we
have shown that it does affect the phosphororylation of
the cell membrane by activating cyclic AMP dependent
protein kinase.

M. W. Bitensky: May I comment on this? I would like
to say first that according to prevailing dogma, cyclic
AMP functions within the cell where it arises, I think

that this is reasonable because of the fact that cyclic
AMP although at a high concentration outside is apt to
reach very small concentrations inside. Now I think it's
interesting that one can get activity with Sepharose linked
cyclic nucleotides. Three alternatives that have been
considered for the mode of action dibutyryl cyclic AMP are
that it can inhibit phosphodiesterase, that the buytryl
groups could be removed so that it becomes cyclic AMP or
that it directly activates protein kinase. Villar-Palasi
has shown that the dibutyryl cyclic AMP, can activate
protein kinase with a K_a of 10^{-5} M compared to a K_a for
cyclic AMP of 10^{-7} M. N^6-monobutyryl cyclic AMP is about
as effective as cyclic AMP ($K_a = 2 \times 10^{-7}$ M). So that
I would say that the central outlines of the dogma that
cyclic nucleotides work by activating protein kinase, and
they work within the cells in which they originate are
preserved. I would not feel free to conclude from the
actions of high concentrations of dibutyryl linked to
Sepharose, that there are receptors at the cell surface.
I think that the central point that you raise with the
data is whether there are cell surface receptors that can
respond to cyclic nucleotides and whether they can function
from the outside of the cell. The fact that they can
function when linked to Sepharose is clear, the fact the
dibutyryl cyclic AMP can function in this way is clear.
The real question is whether there are situations where
cell surfaces are influenced by cyclic AMP on the outside
or whether it always works from within, even though it's
influencing the plasma membrane.

Another problem that has to be considered with the
Sepharose-linked ligands, whether you're dealing with hormones or cyclic nucleotides is the incredible reservoir
capacity of Sepharose and propensity for the linked substance to elute from the Sepharose for days and weeks. So
one has to have really stringent controls showing that
washings from this material are unable to produce these
effects. The solid phase activity of dibutyryl is fine
but I can't yet feel that the very fascinating possibility
of cyclic AMP acting from the outside has been demonstrated.
It certainly has not been excluded. But it hasn't been
proven.

J. Kallos: In two minutes I didn't want to show you too many slides. I just wanted to show you that we can produce not only the effect from the outside, but we can produce it much more effectively. Of course I agree completely that controls for the immobilized AMP studies are extremely crucial because one has to be completely sure that it's acting on the outside. The fact that we produce activity at 100 times lower concentration than with the soluble AMP implies one control, that we are dealing with some different mechanism from the outside than from the inside. I just wanted to raise the possibility that perhaps cyclic AMP can have a dual effect and control cellular processes from the outside as well as intracellularly. Also one can visually demonstrate the receptor sites on the surface.

D. V. K. Murthy, Syntex Research Institute of Biological Sciences: I would like to make one comment on what you said just now, and then I have one question. You mentioned that dibutyryl cyclic AMP (DBcAMP) activates protein kinase. We have investigated this thoroughly and DBcAMP shows about 1% or less of the activity of cAMP (unpublished results; this data was reported at the Pacific Conference on Chemistry and Spectroscopy, San Francisco, October 17, 1972; paper 133). As DBcAMP is relatively unstable, we were not sure whether the activity observed was intrinsic to the molecule or due to probable contamination of cyclic AMP. Therefore, we examined the ability of 2'-O-methyl,2'-O-ethyl and 2'-deoxy derivatives to activate protein kinase, and they all showed less than 0.5% of cyclic AMP activity. Recently, Miller et al. (Biochemistry, 12:1010, 1973) have also shown that DBcAMP and several 2'-O- derivatives possessed less than 1% of the activity of cyclic AMP. These low levels of activity of these derivatives suggest that either DBcAMP possesses extremely low levels of activity or more likely be due to contamination of cyclic AMP or its N^6 monobutyryl derivative.

M. W. Bitensky: Have you seen the paper that I referred to by Villar-Palasi, a recent paper where they very specifically evaluated the efficacy of the butyrated derivatives on purified protein kinase (Biochem. Biophys. Acta <u>321</u> 165-170 (1973)).

D. V. K. Murthy: No, but I would certainly like to see their data. The question that I want to ask you is this. In view of your observation that exposure to light activates phosphodiesterase, have you measured cyclic AMP and cyclic GMP levels under dark and light conditions? If so, did you find any significant differences?

M. W. Bitensky: We have wanted to do that experiment for a long time and we haven't. However, we were just sent a preprint from K. M. Weber at Bochum in Germany (in press in Cytobiologie). They have used histochemical measurements of cyclic AMP phosphodiesterase and found that in the retina there is much more phosphodiesterase in the photo receptors than in any other location. Also they have found very striking differences in activity with light and dark for phosphodiesterase suggesting in fact that there are marked declines in cyclic nucleotide levels under illumination. So this histochemical data supports very nicely the chemical data that we have obtained.

We do not have the direct measurements of content that you have requested. The methodological obstacle to this is that you need to separate the outer segments from the retina before you do the content measurements. You've got to have a way of being certain that you're not changing the nucleotide concentrations during the separation and that's very difficult since separation takes at least 60 minutes. Since the outer segments don't have the machinery for making ATP (or GTP) you can't establish a viable system in vitro as you can for many other tissues.

W. Lands, University of Michigan: I'd like to focus on your mixing experiments. You indicated the activation of the diesterase occurs extremely rapidly and it only takes small amounts of added activator to do this. The two features about the activator that I'm interested in relate to whether it's communicating through an aqueous medium or through a membrane or lipo-protein medium. First, could the small bits of activating material that are put in exert their action through a dialysis membrane in the same tube? Secondly, if you use this, and you activate a system and then you use your differential heat treatment to destroy all the diesterase that's been activated, is there any remaining activating capacity left?

Is it a consumable ability or is it more a more permanent capacity for activation?

M. W. *Bitensky*: You've touched on I think one of the most peculiar features of the system. Because what we are describing would appear to be a very rapid reaction which depends on particle-particle interaction. We have looked for a soluble communicator for these reasons. We haven't used the dialysis membrane design that you described, although it's a good one, and we plan to. The only one that we've tried is the simplest, and that is to take a large quantity of the membranes, illuminate them, and then sediment them so that the membranes are removed and see whether a concentrated supernatant from that preparation could then influence the phosphodiesterase activity in unilluminated membranes. This would be a reasonably sensitive way to look for the release of some soluble intermediate.

W. *Lands*: How about the consumability of it?

M. W. *Bitensky*: Let me finish this one. There is no evidence whatsoever that we are successful in releasing such a soluble intermediate. Now, as far as the consumability is concerned, we haven't done that experiment either but the evidence suggests that the activator is very stable, that once you produce the activator, that it's activating properties persist. For instance, it is absolutely rock stable in the freezer and it is absolutely rock stable in under the conditions of the assay.

B. F. *Erlanger*: In reference to your reluctance to accept your own data about k_{cat} increasing. We've been working with a series of systems which mimic photoresponsive systems that appear in nature. In essence, we've been using photochromic effector molecules to activate membranes, for example the electrogenic membrane of the electric eel, and also to activate and inhibit enzymes. In one of the enzyme systems, we observe an increase in k_{cat} without an increase in K_m. You shouldn't therefore, be reluctant to consider this as a viable possibility.

J. Wolff, National Institutes of Health: I have two questions referring to previous questions. Are you not worried about the rather enormous discrepancy between your actual concentration of cyclic nucleotides and the K_m? Is the dissipation of the activated state, in fact, going to be sufficiently rapid to return it to some sort of a ground state for photic events to happen?

M. W. Bitensky: I don't understand the first question so help me with that again. But let me answer the second one. The dissipation, we don't really have yet adequate data to measure the dissipation of the activated state. The reason for this is that in the normal state of events with the normal anatomic relationships retained, rhodopsin is very rapidly regenerated after illumination and lots of things occur which don't occur in our system. In other words in our isolated membrane vesicles following illumination we don't get regeneration of 11 cis-retinal and the recovery of the native state, so I can't answer that. Now, what about this preponderence of one to another, I didn't get that?

J. Wolff: The expected concentration of the cyclic nucleotides will be in the 10 nanomolar range, but your K_m is in the millimolar range; will you get sufficient rates to get anything?

M. W. Bitensky: We have run these reactions with the expected concentrations of cyclic nucleotides. I would not say nanomolar, I would say 10^{-7} molar, and under those conditions we get very rapid hydrolysis.

STUDIES ON THE MEMBRANES OF HUMAN NORMAL AND LEUKEMIC LYMPHOCYTES

C. W. ABELL, R. R. FRITZ, R. A. NOVAK and T. M. MONAHAN
Division of Biochemistry
Department of Human Biological Chemistry and Genetics
The University of Texas Medical Branch, Galveston

INTRODUCTION

Peripheral blood lymphocytes represent a unique model for the study of the conversion of cells from the resting to the dividing state. When these cells are freshly isolated, they are presumed to be under physiological control since they are quiescent. In culture, lymphocytes exhibit protein and RNA synthesis but not cellular DNA synthesis unless they are challenged with a mitogen or antigen. A wide variety of plant lectins, some antigens, and a few small molecular weight compounds stimulate mitotic division when added to lymphocytes (1, 2). Using such agents, it is possible to study how mitogenesis is initiated, what components on the cell surface are involved, and what early events are critical to the progression of cells into the dividing state. Furthermore, by employing lymphocytes from healthy human donors and from patients with chronic lymphocytic leukemia (CLL), it is possible to examine biochemical properties that may be different between these two cell types.

One method of studying cell membranes in resting and dividing cells is to determine the activity of specific membrane bound enzymes. The hormone sensitive enzyme adenylate cyclase is a component of cell membranes (3). This enzyme catalyzes the synthesis of cyclic AMP, an intracellular mediator of various physiological processes. Cyclic AMP is cleaved to AMP-5' by one or more phosphodiesterases. Recent evidence suggests that cyclic AMP may play a role in regulating division in lymphocytes (4) and other cells (5). Thus, by a comparison of the cyclic AMP system in normal and CLL lymphocytes, we can examine if differences exist between these two cell types.

RESULTS AND DISCUSSION

Comparative Studies on Cyclic AMP in Normal and Leukemic Lymphocytes

Previous studies (6, 7) in our laboratory have demonstrated that normal and CLL lymphocytes differ in their time of onset of DNA synthesis and in their sensitivity to drugs or compounds (isoproterenol, cyclic AMP, and theophylline) which presumably raise the intracellular levels of cyclic AMP. More recently, the levels of cyclic AMP and glycogen and the activities of glycogen phosphorylase and cyclic AMP phosphodiesterase in normal and CLL lymphocytes in the resting and mitogen-stimulated states have been studied (8). The results of these comparisons indicate the following:

(a) CLL cells undergo maximal DNA synthesis 5 to 7 days after stimulation with PHA, whereas normal cells respond maximally 3 to 4 days after PHA addition;

(b) CLL cells are more sensitive to inhibition by isoproterenol, cyclic AMP, and dibutyryl cyclic AMP than normal cells;

(c) CLL cells contain approximately 3-fold higher levels of glycogen than normal cells in the resting state;

(d) Glycogen phosphorylase activities are lower in CLL cells than in normal cells following mitogenic stimulation;

228

(e) CLL cells have 2 to 4-fold lower levels of cyclic AMP than normal cells in the resting state;

(f) and Cyclic AMP phosphodiesterase activities are higher in CLL cells than in normal cells.

Collectively, these observations demonstrate that the physiological participation of the cyclic AMP system differs in these two cell types.

In recent years, however, it has become clear that the small lymphocyte population of the peripheral blood consists of two major populations, T and B cells (9, 10, 11). In normal lymphocytes the T cell comprises 80 to 90% of the total lymphocyte population. In contrast, lymphocytes from the peripheral blood of patients with CLL are predominantly B cells with known surface immunoglobulins (12, 13). Thus, the biochemical comparisons that have been found are presumed to be between T cells from healthy donors and B cells from patients with CLL. The differences that have been delineated may therefore represent ones between two normal cell types rather than differences between a normal and "leukemic" population of cells. Comparisons of cyclic AMP levels in B cells isolated from normal donors with those in lymphocytes obtained from patients with CLL may resolve this question. The interpretation of these results, however, might be further complicated by the presence of several sub types of either T or B cells in which cyclic AMP levels may differ.

Periodate Stimulation of Lymphocytes
One of the new agents for the investigation of the interaction of mitogens with cells is sodium periodate (14, 15, 16). The use of this small molecular weight compound has the advantage that it can be completely removed shortly after cells are exposed to it. Sodium periodate is relatively non-specific, however, in that it may oxidize a variety of cellular components. Nevertheless, conditions may be selected where oxidation is thought to occur primarily at exposed sites on the cell surface. Under these conditions, the mechanism by which cells respond to

changes on their surface and if they recognize alterations induced by sodium periodate on neighboring cells may be studied.

Conditions Used for Periodate Oxidation

Previous studies by Parker et al. (15, 17) demonstrated that
the addition of sodium periodate at room temperature for 10
minutes markedly stimulated DNA synthesis in peripheral blood
lymphocytes. Under their conditions, sodium periodate gave
maximal DNA synthesis at a concentration of 4×10^{-3}M. As
shown in Figure 1, we observed a similar stimulation when
normal lymphocytes (purified by passage through glass wool
columns or by ficoll-hypaque gradient centrifugation) were
treated with sodium periodate over a range of 10^{-3}M to 10^{-2}M.
Maximal DNA synthesis was obtained when a periodate concentration of 3×10^{-3}M was used, whereas, the rate of synthesis
was appreciably less at higher concentrations of the mitogen.
Even at the optimum concentration, however, periodate-stimulated DNA synthesis was only approximately 25% of that obtained with PHA. Furthermore, treatment with sodium
periodate resulted in a significant loss of cell viability and cell
number during subsequent culturing. In an attempt to improve
conditions, cells were incubated with sodium periodate for 10
minutes at 4°C, washed in medium at room temperature to
remove the mitogen, and then resuspended in complete medium.
As shown in Figure 1, the extent of DNA synthesis was greater
under these conditions. Maximal activity was observed at a
sodium periodate concentration of approximately 5×10^{-3}M
(although higher concentrations are not shown in this figure).
The response of lymphocytes to periodate was about 75% of that
to PHA at 48 hours, and these cells remained approximately
90% viable for several days following treatment.

Figure 2 illustrates the response of CLL lymphocytes as a
function of periodate concentration. These lymphocytes also
demonstrated maximal DNA synthesis at a periodate concentration of about 5×10^{-3}M.

Figure 3 shows the response of normal lymphocytes to
sodium periodate as a function of time. As observed for PHA-

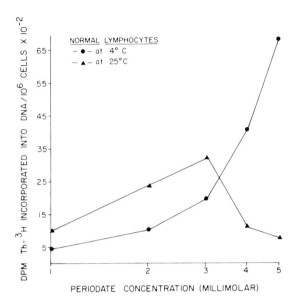

Fig. 1. Stimulation of normal lymphocytes with different concentrations of periodate at two different temperatures. Peripheral blood was obtained from healthy donors, platelets were removed by controlled clotting and lymphocytes were separated on ficoll-hypaque density gradients. The isolated lymphocytes were washed and resuspended in phosphate buffered saline (PBS) at a concentration of 12.5×10^6 cells/ml and then treated with $NaIO_4$ for 10 minutes at the appropriate concentration and temperature. The cells were then washed, resuspended at a concentration of 2×10^6 cells/ml in complete Mc Coy's media containing 10% (V/V) autologous serum. DNA synthesis was determined at 48 hours using the incorporation of thymidine-[3]H.

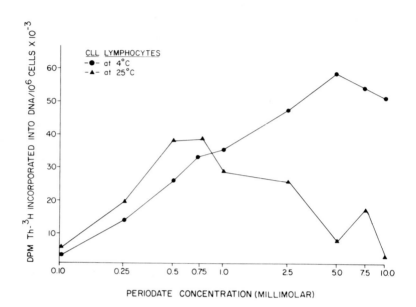

Fig. 2. Stimulation of CLL lymphocytes with varying concentrations of periodate at two different temperatures. Peripheral blood lymphocytes from CLL patients were prepared and treated as described in Figure 1. The white blood count (WBC) of these patients ranged from 30,000 to 40,000 with a range of 80 to 95% lymphocytes. DNA synthesis was determined at 96 and 120 hours.

stimulated cells, little or no incorporation of thymidine into DNA was observed for 24 hours. DNA synthesis began subsequently and reached a maximum at 48 hours. In contrast to the pattern observed with PHA, however, DNA synthesis in the sodium periodate-stimulated cultures was reduced at 72 hours to less than 25% of the activity observed at 48 hours. Nevertheless, cell numbers and DNA content increased by 25 to 30% which indicates that some lymphocytes in the culture divided at least once. In PHA stimulated cultures, a 1.5 to 2-fold increase in DNA content and cell number usually occurs within 4 days.

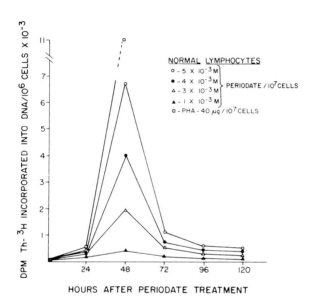

Fig. 3. DNA synthesis in normal lymphocytes stimulated with different concentrations of NaIO$_4$. Cells were prepared as described in Figure 1 and pulse labelled with thymidine-^{3}H (0.5 uC/ml for 2 hours) at the times indicated.

In order to investigate differences between normal and leukemic cells, lymphocytes from patients with CLL were isolated, purified on ficoll-hypaque gradients, and treated with sodium periodate under the conditions described for normal lymphocytes. As shown in Figure 4, CLL lymphocytes responded to periodate more extensively than to PHA, and the extent of DNA synthesis was greater than that observed in sodium periodate-stimulated cultures of normal lymphocytes. The con-

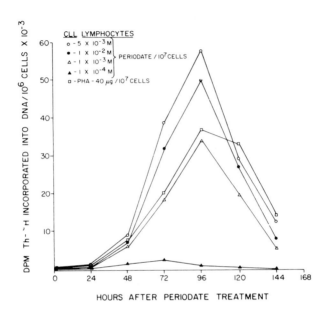

Fig. 4. DNA synthesis in CLL lymphocytes stimulated with different concentrations of NaIO$_4$. Cells were prepared as described in Figure 1 and pulse labelled with thymidine-^{3}H (0.5 uC/ml for 2 hours) at the times indicated.

centration of periodate required to give maximal DNA synthesis was 5 x 10^{-3}M which is approximately the same concentration found with normal lymphocytes. Unlike normal lymphocytes, however, the response to sodium periodate was maximal at 96 hours after addition of the mitogen rather than at 48 hours, when little activity was detected. A delayed peak of DNA synthesis in CLL lymphocytes was also found when PHA is used as a mitogen (6). Our observation of the response of CLL lymphocytes to sodium periodate is in contrast to a study by Parker et al. (18) who did not obtain stimulation.

Effects of Sodium Borohydride and Enzymes on the Mitogenic
Activity of Sodium Periodate

In order to examine further the biological nature of the
mitogenic activity of sodium periodate, stimulated lymphocytes
were treated sequentially with enzymes which specifically cleave
sialic acid or glycopeptides from the membrane or with sodium
borohydride. Table 1 shows the results of such studies. When
lymphocytes were stimulated with PHA, approximately 12,200
DPM, 39,300 DPM and 52,500 DPM of thymidine-^{3}H were incorporated into DNA (per 10^6 cells) at 48, 72, and 96 hours,
respectively, after addition of the mitogen. These figures are
arbitrarily considered as 100% response. When lymphocytes
were treated with neuraminidase for 60 minutes, washed to
remove the enzyme, and incubated in fresh media, little or no
stimulation of DNA synthesis was observed. Alternatively, when
neuraminidase treated lymphocytes were stimulated with PHA,
responses of 130, 75, and 58% were observed within 48, 72, and
96 hours, respectively. These results indicate that treatment
with neuraminidase under conditions which remove more than
50% of the surface sialic acid (14, 19) does not prevent lymphocytes from responding to PHA. Although the sialic acid moiety
in the glycoprotein may not be required for the mitogenic activity
of PHA, alternate explanations are that "sialic acid repair"
occurred or that new receptor sites were exposed on the surface
of the cell.

When lymphocytes were treated with trypsin for one hour to
remove glycopeptides from the cell surface (20), washed and
resuspended in complete medium, little or no stimulation of DNA
synthesis occurred. The addition of PHA to trypsin-treated lymphocytes gave responses of 155, 141, and 70% of the control at
48, 72, and 96 hours, respectively. Since glycopeptides are
presumed to be involved in the mitogenic activity of PHA,
possible explanations of these results are that the essential
receptor glycopeptides were resynthesized as a prerequisite to
the initiation of mitogenesis by PHA or that the cell topography
was altered thus exposing new binding sites.

Effects of PHA, Periodate, Borohydride, and Enzymes on DNA Synthesis in Normal Lymphocytes

	Th-^{3}H Incorporated into DNA/10^6 Cells		
	48 hrs.	72 hrs.	96 hrs.
	%	%	%
PHA	100	100	100
Neuraminidase	2	2	1
Neuraminidase + PHA	141	79	58
Trypsin	2	1	1
Trypsin + PHA	152	141	70
$NaIO_4$	75	11	2
$NaIO_4$ + PHA	81	63	69
$NaIO_4$ + Neuraminidase	43	8	2
$NaIO_4$ + Neuraminidase + PHA	76	53	51
$NaIO_4$ + Trypsin	29	13	2
$NaIO_4$ + Trypsin + PHA	60	49	72
$NaIO_4$ + $NaBH_4$	9	5	2
$NaIO_4$ + $NaBH_4$ + PHA	86	95	98
$NaIO_4$ + $NaBH_4$ + Neuraminidase	12	8	3
$NaIO_4$ + $NaBH_4$ + Neuraminidase + PHA	63	56	73
$NaIO_4$ + $NaBH_4$ + Trypsin	2	2	2
$NaIO_4$ + $NaBH_4$ + Trypsin + PHA	75	92	115

Table 1. Cells were treated sequentially with the agents indicated above. The conditions for the treatment of 10^7 cells/ml phosphate buffered saline (PBS) were: neuraminidase (50 units, 60 min.), trypsin (25 μg, 60 min.) $NaIO_4$ (5 x 10^{-3}M, 10 min., 4°C), $NaBH_4$ (5 x 10^{-3}M, 30 min., 4°C), and PHA (40 μg,

continuous) in media. DNA synthesis was determined using thymidine-^{3}H (SA = 2.0 C/mmole, 0.5 μC/ml), 2 hour pulse for 2 x 10^6 cells/ml. The activities in the PHA-stimulated cells were 12,200, 39,300, and 52,500 DPM at 48, 72, and 96 hours, respectively. These values were arbitrarily considered as 100% response. All determinations were performed in duplicate and varied within $\pm$ 10%.

The effects of these enzymes on periodate and/or PHA-stimulated lymphocytes were also examined. Lymphocytes responded to periodate to approximately 75% of the PHA response within 48 hours. As indicated previously, these cells undergo maximal DNA synthesis at 48 hours but have a much reduced synthetic rate at 72 and 96 hours. Cells that were treated with periodate and PHA gave approximately the same response as did periodate alone at 48 hours; however, at 72 hours, periodate and PHA additions resulted in a 63% response. Since the PHA and sodium periodate induced stimulations were not additive at 48 hours, it may be presumed that the receptors for these two mitogens are the same. If this is true, the stimulation observed at 72 and 96 hours with PHA, but not sodium periodate, may reflect repeated cell division in the PHA lymphocyte cultures. This concept suggests that a mitogen must be present for each round of DNA replication. Alternate explanations are that the PHA and periodate sites are different or that different sub populations of lymphocytes are stimulated. Our present studies do not allow us to distinguish between these possibilities.

When cells were treated with periodate and then with neuraminidase, DNA synthesis was reduced to 43% of the PHA control and about 60% of the periodate control at 48 hours. These results may indicate that events which are prerequisites for the onset of DNA synthesis were only partially initiated prior to neuraminidase treatment. If this is true, lymphocytes may require a finite period of time in their oxidized state for complete activation. Treatment of cells sequentially with periodate, neuraminidase, and PHA gave a response at 48 hours

237

similar to that elucidated by periodate alone or periodate plus PHA.

Treatment of periodate-stimulated lymphocytes with trypsin resulted in a pronounced inhibition of DNA synthesis. Nevertheless, when these cells were then treated with PHA, DNA synthesis approached that observed in the lymphocytes stimulated with periodate plus PHA. The fact that treatment of cells with trypsin (following periodate stimulation) significantly reduces the response is a further indication that events critical to the conversion of resting cells to dividing ones occur soon after mitogenic stimulation.

The effects of reduction by sodium borohydride on periodate-stimulated cells were determined. Following periodate oxidation of lymphocytes, treatment with sodium borohydride almost completely inhibited DNA synthesis in these cultures. Sequential treatment with periodate, borohydride, and PHA, however, elucidated a full response (95% of the PHA control). These results clearly demonstrate that oxidation and reduction of cells under the conditions described do not produce irreversible damage.

Cells treated with periodate, borohydride, and neuraminidase show little response, whereas, when these cells are subsequently treated with PHA, 56 to 73% response was subsequently obtained. Furthermore, cells which were treated sequentially with periodate, borohydride, and trypsin and then stimulated with PHA, elucidated a complete response.

Oxidation and Reductive Labelling of Neuraminidase and Trypsin Sensitive Residues

In order to determine the specificity of the oxidation and reduction of specific components of cells, studies were performed with sodium periodate and sodium borohydride-^{3}H under the same conditions described previously for biological activity. The cells were then treated with neuraminidase to determine how much of the label which had been introduced into the cell surface was removed. As shown in Figure 5, treatment with neuramini-

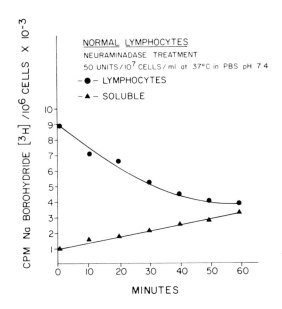

Fig. 5. Release of cell surface structures labelled with $NaBH_4$-^3H. Normal peripheral blood lymphocytes were prepared and oxidized as described in Figure 1. The cells were then resuspended in PBS and reduced with $NaBH_4$-^3H at a concentration of 5 x $10^{-3}M$ (cell concentration 11.5 x 10^6 cells/ml) for 30 minutes at 4°C. These cells were then split into two groups and treated as indicated on the graph with either neuraminidase or trypsin (see Figure 6).

dase for 60 minutes removed approximately 80% of the label which had been introduced into residues of the cell. In view of this observation, and since it has been shown that neuraminidase removes the exposed sialic acid in the membrane (19), we suggest that sialic acid is oxidized by periodate. A recent study by Liao et al. (21) on the periodate oxidation of erythrocytes supports this possibility.

Exposure of periodate oxidized-and borohydride-^{3}H reduced lymphocytes to trypsin resulted in the removal of approximately 80% of the label (Figure 6). These results coupled with the biological activity induced by such agents also suggest that sialic acid containing glycopeptides exposed on the cell surface are receptors of periodate treatment.

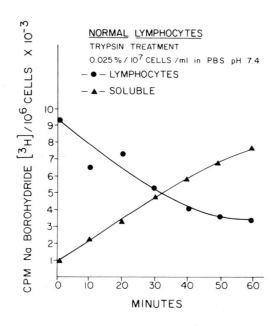

Fig. 6. See legend to Figure 5.

Autologous Mixed Lymphocyte Cultures

How cells recognize changes that arise in their surface or upon the surface of neighboring cells was investigated using the procedure designed in Figure 7. This procedure is similar to the classical mixed lymphocyte cultures (22) but here uses autologous cells. Peripheral blood lymphocytes from healthy donors were resolved on ficoll-hypaque gradients and were then divided into two groups. One group was treated with mitomycin

Autologous Mixed Lymphocyte Cultures

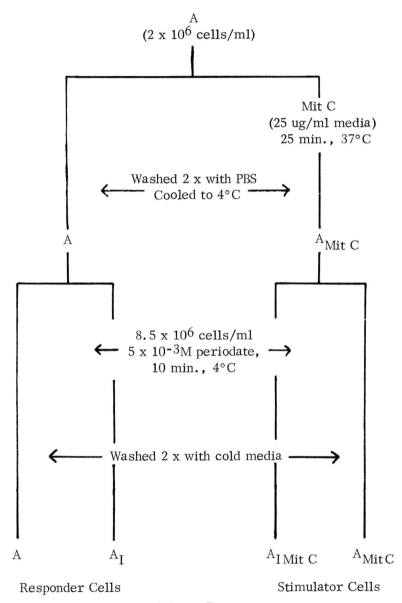

Figure 7

C for 25 minutes at 37°C to prevent DNA synthesis. These cells and the controls were then washed two times with PBS and cooled to 4°C. The control and the mitomycin C treated cells were separated into two sub groups. One sub group remained un-treated and is designated as the responder cell (A). Another sub group was designated as A_{Mit_3C}. The two other sub groups of cells were treated with 5 x 10^{-3}M periodate for 10 minutes at 4°C, were then washed two times with cold complete media as were the controls, and were designated as A_I, which is the mitogen treated cell, and $A_{I\,Mit\,C}$ which represents the stimulator cells. Thus, by a combination of the cells that have been treated as indicated, we can determine if lymphocytes recognize changes that have been introduced into the surface by periodate oxidation (Table 2).

The results show that the untreated responder cells A, have little activity alone but exhibit extensive DNA synthesis when mixed with stimulator cells ($A_{I\,Mit\,C}$). Maximal activity was obtained when cells were mixed at a ratio of approximately 1 : 1. This is observed more easily when the counts contributed by $A_{I\,Mit\,C}$ (approximately 8% of A_I) are subtracted from the values obtained in the mixture. The activity observed in these types of autologous mixed lymphocyte cultures was usually 25 to 30% of the activity obtained in the periodate stimulated cells (A_I).

These studies clearly demonstrate that lymphocytes, which have not been exposed to a mitogen, may be stimulated by cells which have been treated with periodate.

One possible mechanism by which responder cells are stimulated to divide by stimulator cells is through the release or production of a lymphocyte growth factor. In order to determine whether such a factor exists in these cultures, the following observations were made (Table 3). Periodate-stimulated cells showed extensive activity at 48 hours whereas non-stimulated cells demonstrated little incorporation of thymidine-^{3}H into DNA. When media (which contains no residual periodate) obtained from a 24 hour periodate-stimulated culture was added to non-stimu-lated cells (A),they demonstrated extensive DNA synthesis with-

TABLE 2

Effect of Stimulator Cells on Responder Cells in Autologous
Mixed Lymphocyte Cultures

Cell Type	Number of Responder Cells	Number of Stimulator Cells	CPM Th-^{3}H Incorporated into DNA ($\pm$SD)	
			Total culture CPM	Net CPM/10^6 responder cells
A	7.5×10^5	0	962 ± 31	
A$_I$	1.0×10^6	0	$27,300 \pm 483$	
A$_I$ Mit C	0	1.0×10^6	$2,180 \pm 112$	
A + A$_I$ Mit C	7.5×10^5	0.50×10^6	$5,250 \pm 230$	5,560
A + A$_I$ Mit C	7.5×10^5	0.62×10^6	$6,180 \pm 124$	6,420
A + A$_I$ Mit C	7.5×10^5	1.25×10^6	$6,500 \pm 228$	5,030
A + A$_I$ Mit C	7.5×10^5	2.5×10^6	$6,180 \pm 173$	974
A + A$_I$ Mit C	7.5×10^5	5.0×10^6	$5,320 \pm 285$	-0-

Table 2. Normal untreated lymphocytes (A) were mixed with various numbers of periodate-stimulated, mitomycin C blocked lymphocytes from the same donor and cultured in a final volume of 1 ml. Thymidine-^{3}H incorporation into DNA was measured after 48 hours. Total culture counts were corrected for residual DNA synthesis in A$_I$ Mit C.

TABLE 3

Production of Lymphocyte Growth Factor

Cell Type	Number of Responder Cells	Additions	Time in Culture	CPM Th-^{3}H Incorporated into DNA/10^6 cells ($\pm$SD)
A_I	1.0×10^6	None	24 hrs.	$2,400 \pm 154$
A_I	1.0×10^6	None	48 hrs.	$27,300 \pm 483$
A	0.75×10^6	None	24 hrs.	545 ± 20
A	0.75×10^6	None	48 hrs.	962 ± 31
A	0.75×10^6	A_I Media	24 hrs.	$3,820 \pm 66$
A	0.75×10^6	A_I Media	48 hrs.	$15,000 \pm 900$

Table 3. Normal lymphocytes (A) were suspended in media obtained from periodate-stimulated cells that had been in culture for 24 hours. The conditions of the periodate treatment were as described previously (5 x 10^{-3}M for 10 min. at 4°C). Thymidine-^{3}H incorporation into DNA was measured subsequently at the times indicated.

244

in 48 hours (approximately 50% of the periodate treated control).
These results clearly implicate a lymphocyte growth factor,
which when produced or released from the mitogen-stimulated
cells, influences the DNA synthetic activity in neighboring cells.

Summary

Various parameters of the cyclic AMP system have been
compared between normal and CLL lymphocytes. CLL lymphocytes are more sensitive to additions of isoproterenol or cyclic
AMP, and contain lower intracellular levels of cyclic AMP.
Glycogen phosphorylase and cyclic AMP phosphodiesterase,
which are regulated by cyclic AMP, gave activities that are
consistent with the levels of the cyclic nucleotide in each cell
type. These results suggest that the cyclic AMP system is
physiologically different in normal and CLL lymphocytes.
Whether this is a difference between B and T populations of lymphocytes or between a true "leukemic" population and normal
lymphocytes is presently unknown.

Under mild conditions, sodium periodate stimulates some
lymphocytes to undergo DNA synthesis and mitotic division.
Lymphocytes obtained from healthy donors and from patients
with CLL participate in this reaction.

The mitogenic activity of periodate in normal lymphocytes is
essentially completely blocked by treatment with sodium borohydride. By the use of labelled sodium borohydride, it was
found that approximately 80% of the label that was introduced into
the periodate oxidized cell surface was susceptible to cleavage
by neuraminidase and trypsin. Consequently, we propose that
periodate oxidation occurs on glycopeptides containing sialic acid.

By means of autologous mixed lymphocyte cultures, it was
demonstrated that untreated lymphocytes respond to changes that
have been introduced into periodate treated cells. The precise
mechanism of this stimulation is unknown but a growth promoting
factor, that is either produced or released from periodate
treated cells, stimulates DNA synthesis in untreated lymphocytes.

245

REFERENCES

(1) P. C. Nowell. Cancer Res. 20 (1960) 462.

(2) H. L. Cooper. Drugs and the Cell Cycle (Academic Press, New York, 1973) p. 137.

(3) G. A. Robison, R. W. Butcher and E. W. Sutherland. Cyclic AMP (Academic Press, New York, 1971) p. 22.

(4) J. W. Smith, A. L. Steiner, W. M. Newberry and C. W. Parker. J. Clin. Invest. 50 (1971) 432.

(5) C. W. Abell and T. M. Monahan. J. Cell Biol. 59 (1973) 549.

(6) C. W. Abell, C. W. Kamp and L. D. Johnson. Cancer Res. 30 (1970) 717.

(7) L. D. Johnson and C. W. Abell. Cancer Res. 30 (1970) 2718.

(8) C. W. Abell, N. W. Marchand and T. M. Monahan. Cancer Res. Submitted, 1974.

(9) N. B. Everett and R. W. Tyler. Formation and Destruction of Blood Cells (Lippincott, Philadelphia, 1970) p. 264.

(10) P. Heller, N. Bhoopalam, V. J. Yakulis and N. Costea. Clin. Exp. Immunol. 9 (1971) 637.

(11) N. I. Abdan. J. Immunol. 107 (1971) 1637.

(12) C. Bianco, R. Patrick and V. N. Nussenzweig. J. Exp. Med. 132 (1970) 702.

(13) H. M. Grey, E. Rabellino and B. Pirofsky. J. Clin. Invest. 50 (1971) 2368.

(14) A. Novogrodsky and E. Katchalski. Proc. Nat. Acad. Sci. 69 (1972) 3207.

(15) J. W. Parker, R. L. O'Brien, R. J. Lukes, J. Steiner and P. Paolilli. Immunol. Commun. 1 (1972) 263.

(16) M. M. Zatz, A. L. Goldstein, O. O. Blumenfeld and A. White. Nature, New Biol. 240 (1972) 252.

(17) J. W. Parker, R. L. O'Brien, J. Steiner and P. Paolilli. Exp. Cell Res. 78 (1973) 279.

(18) J. W. Parker, R. L. O'Brien, R. J. Lukes and J. Steiner. Lancet 1 (1972) 103.

(19) P. K. Ray and R. L. Simmons. Cancer Res. 33 (1973) 936.

(20) S. Kornfeld and R. Kornfeld. Proc. Nat. Acad. Sci. 63 (1969) 1439.

(21) T. H. Liao, P. M. Gallop and O. O. Blumenfeld. J. Biol. Chem. 248 (1973) 8247.

(22) F. H. Bach and N. K. Voynow. Science 153 (1966) 545.

ACKNOWLEDGMENT

This investigation was supported by USPHS Research Grant CA-14525 from the National Cancer Institute, NIH.

DISCUSSION

K. Muench, University of Miami: I have some questions on the periodate treatment. Have you shown that there is actual consumption of the periodate, for example with the 5 millimolar periodate giving maximal response? Is that periodate entirely converted to iodate, and if so, does iodate have any effect?

C.W. Abell, University of Texas: No, we have not measured the consumption of periodate directly or the effect of iodate. Of course, the experiments in which cells were treated with periodate followed by reduction with tritium labeled sodium borohydride, and then the label was removed with neuraminidase or trypsin, indicated that there are some sites on the cell surface that are oxidized with periodate. Also, since reduction with borohydride prevents periodate-stimulated DNA synthesis, the cells must remain in the oxidized state for a finite period of time.

K. Muench: But in terms of quantitation?

C.W. Abell: Approximately 80% of the label was removed by neuraminidase or trypsin treatment of the cells that were oxidized and reduced with ^{3}H-borohydride. We have not determined directly the amount of periodate that reacted with components on the cell surface.

K. Muench: At what pH do you do the periodate oxidation?

C.W. Abell: This was done at 7.4.

K. Muench: Is any sugar present in the medium?

C.W. Abell: No, the lymphocytes were treated with periodate in phosphate buffered saline.

K. Muench: And finally, do you have a measure of the percentage of CLL cells in the culture which respond by cell division?

C.W. Abell: No, not with periodate stimulation. When PHA is added to CLL lymphocytes, however, 30 to 50% of the cells respond within 7 days. In comparison to PHA, periodate apparently stimulated a similar percentage of lymphocytes. The growth fraction is currently being determined by autoradiography.

R.C. Leif, Papanicolaou Cancer Research Institute: These experiments are presumably all on lymphocytes. How did you separate the lymphocytes and how did you ascertain whether you had lymphocytes?

C.W. Abell: They were separated either on ficoll-hypaque gradients or on glass wool columns. The populations obtained were examined microscopically and were deemed to be small lymphocytes by classical staining techniques.

R.C. Leif: Did the Ficoll-hypaque isolated cells have any monocytes as a contaminant?

C.W. Abell: Yes, all of the preparations had monocytes present, however, the lymphocytes comprised about 95 to 98% of the population. The remainder of the population was primarily monocytes. This is why I mentioned in the talk that we do not know the role of monocytes in the release of the lymphocyte growth factor.

M.Z. Atassi, Wayne State University: I have a question concerning the periodate oxidation, the effect you observed in the experiments with periodate and then periodate plus PHA, periodate plus trypsin, periodate plus neuraminidase. I wondered if this effect cannot be explained adequately by the action of periodate on PHA, on trypsin, or on neuraminidase leading to their inactivation. Some years ago we showed (Biochem. J., 167, 102, 478) that the action of periodate on proteins resulted in the oxidation of several amino acids in the primary structure. Of these, after 3 hours of oxidation at 0 degrees the following amino acids oxidized most rapidly: methionine followed by tryptophan, followed by tyrosine. Histidine was oxidized at longer durations of reaction (6 hours). This may in fact be one of the reasons why inactivation of the enzymes employed in your system is completely prevented by the action of sodium borohydride. I wonder if you could comment on that.

C.W. Abell: All of the treatments of cells were performed sequentially in phosphate buffered saline. For example, lymphocytes were treated with periodate for 10 minutes in phosphate buffered saline, and then the cells were added to complete media and washed 2 times before subsequent treatment.

M.Z. Atassi: In other words excess periodate was removed before you added neuraminidase.

C.W. Abell: Yes.

S. Ristow, University of Minnesota: I'd like to have you speculate on the nature of your growth factor. Do you think its like the transfer factor described by Lawrence or immune RNA as described by Gottlieb?

C.W. Abell: It is too early to speculate on this. We have carried out only a very few experiments on the chemical nature of the lymphocyte growth factor, so I'd rather defer an answer to that.

J. Jaroszewski, Naval Medical Research Institute: It has been recently shown by Steffen and Jondal (personal communication) that human B lymphocytes have longer cell cycle times than human T lymphocytes, which seems to be in line with your findings. However, it is my experience that, similarly as Andersson, Sjöberg and Möller have found for mouse B lymphocytes (Transplantation Rev., 1972), conditions for stimulation of human

B lymphocytes differ greatly from those necessary to stimulate human T lymphocytes. If you have suboptimal stimulation of lymphocytes, you've got different kinetics of the response. Can you exclude that in your case you did not use suboptimal dose of mitogen for stimulating leukemic lymphocytes and this could explain the difference in kinetics?

C.W. Abell: I doubt it because we have used a wide concentration range of the mitogen and measured DNA synthesis at many points in time. The delay in the time of maximal DNA synthesis in CLL lymphocytes, when compared to normal lymphocytes, is more likely due to either basic differences in B and T cells or to the leukemic nature of the CLL cell.

J. Whitehead, San Francisco, Calif.: I was wondering if the neuraminidase or trypsin treatment of the cells could have blocked transport of tritiated thymidine into the cell rather than blocking DNA synthesis.

C.W. Abell: That is a possibility since we did not measure pool sizes. Nevertheless, we did measure DNA content and cell number in periodate treated lymphocytes and found an increase of about 30% in both. Thus, the stimulation observed is clearly not simply a transport phenomenon. In the case of trypsin and neuraminidase treated cells, the metabolic activity of the lymphocytes is qualitatively small, indicating that a change in transport is not responsible for the presumed decrease in DNA synthesis.

R.W. Jeanloz, Massachusetts General Hospital: Have you considered the possibility of formaldehyde being released and combining immediately with the protein part, with the free amino groups of proteins? Have you made a similar treatment with a dilute solution of formaldehyde?

C.W. Abell: We have considered that possibility. Those experiments are currently being performed.

NUCLEAR MAGNETIC RESONANCE STUDIES OF MEMBRANES
OF NORMAL AND CANCER CELLS

R.E. BLOCK AND G.P. MAXWELL
Papanicolaou Cancer Research Institute
Miami, Florida 33123

G.L. IRVIN, J.L. HUDSON AND D.L. PRUDHOMME
Veteran's Administration Hospital
Miami, Florida   33136

Abstract- A preliminary study has been made of the 100 MHz
proton nuclear magnetic resonance (NMR) spectra of
packed intact EL-4 ascites tumor and normal mouse
spleen cells as well as EL-4 plasma membrane preparations. The intact cells have lipid resonances
similar to those seen in lipid extracts. The lipid
resonances of the EL-4 cells show variation in
intensity with changes of osmolarity or inclusion
of calcium chloride in the incubation media. The
lipid resonances of the EL-4 cells show line
broadening upon the addition of concanavallin A.
The observation of these effects combined with the
similarity of the EL-4 membrane spectra to those
from intact EL-4 cells suggests that at least a
part of the lipid signals of the intact cells
originate in the plasma membrane. Lower limits of
the diffusion coefficients of the lipid chains in
the mobile lipid fractions of these samples were
estimated from methylene proton linewidths.

INTRODUCTION

Nuclear magnetic resonance (NMR) studies have been
utilized by a number of workers to obtain information
concerning membrane organization. In denaturing or
solubilizing media, the NMR spectra of membranes
generally resemble the sum of fairly well-defined spectra

of the membrane components. However, spectra obtained
from intact membranes or membrane dispersions often tend
to be somewhat broadened and less defined. Peaks in the
latter spectra are often selectively broadened due to
restricted mobility of the corresponding membrane components. Thus information on the composition of membranes
and the mobility of certain membrane components can often
be inferred from the NMR spectra. The accessibility of
membrane components can also be investigated by NMR
studies using probes that broaden or shift spectral
peaks. Some of the biological membranes studied by NMR
to date include: myelin (1-3), erythrocyte ghosts (1),
and sarcoplasmic reticulum (4). However, to our knowledge, no NMR studies have been previously reported on
membranes from tumor cells. In this communication,
a preliminary study of possible techniques for NMR
investigation of membranes from normal spleen cells and
EL-4 tumor cells is presented. Studies of both intact
cells and isolated membranes are reported.

Cerbón (5) showed several years ago that one could
study variations in the state of the lipid components
of living microorganisms by NMR studies of packed cells.
He studied the methyl and methylene proton resonances of
Norcardia asteroides as a function of the osmolarity and
composition of the incubation media. He found that one
could cause increases in the NMR signal intensities by
varying the osmolarity of the incubation media away from
isotonic conditions or by using divalent ions in the
media. He concluded that the signals were changing with
rearrangement of lipids during changes in cellular permeability. In the present study Cerbón's approach of
studying the NMR spectra from intact cells has been
utilized. In addition, isolated plasma membranes
have been studied.

EXPERIMENTAL

Spleens were taken from C57BL/6J female mice 6-8
weeks old. The spleens were placed in tissue culture
media (Hanks solution plus fetal calf serum) until processed further (see Fig. 1) in a batchwise manner. The
spleens were then gently disrupted in a tissue dissociator

SPLEEN CELL PREP.

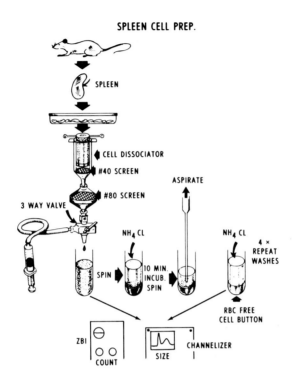

Fig. 1.   An outline of the cell preparation procedure. Use of the syringe and three-way valve allows the cell dissociator to be flushed out without removing the plunger. Spleen white plup is trapped by the #40 mesh screen.

fabricated from a 60 cc. plastic syringe with a # 40 mesh stainless steel screen glued in the barrel. The disrupted tissue was then filtered through a # 80 mesh nylon filter. Cell viability measured by trypan blue dye exclusion remained above 90%. The cells were initially maintained in Dulbecco's phosphate buffered saline (PBS) plus 10% fetal calf serum. In later experi-

255

ments Ca^{++} and Mg^{++} free PBS containing 10% fetal bovine serum and .0025% EDTA adjusted to 307 mOs with NaCl was used to inhibit clumping. The erythrocytes were lysed (6) by three or four treatments consisting of incubation at room temperature for 10 minutes in Tris buffer, pH 7.3, containing 0.16 M NH$_4$Cl. Between incubations the cells were centrifuged in an International PR-2 for five minutes at 30 X g., pelleting the cells while leaving the erythrocyte ghosts in suspension. Cells were counted using a Coulter ZBI and sized using a Coulter Channelizer at each step during the preparation (see Fig. 2). Disappearance of the erythrocyte peak and removal of the cell debris was monitored using the Coulter Channelizer. About 8.5 X 10^7 spleen white cells were obtained per animal.

The EL-4 tumor was originally induced in C57BL mice by the injection of 9,10-dimethyl-1,2-benzanthracene. Gorer (7) originally described the EL-4 as a lymphatic leukemia which later came to resemble a lymphosarcoma. The EL-4 has been carried in our laboratories as a transplantable ascites tumor in C57BL/6J female mice. The tumor was routinely harvested by making an incision into the peritoneal cavity, drawing out the ascitic fluid, and rinsing out the cavity with PBS containing 10% FBS. The average yield per animal was 5 X 10^8 cells. The tumor cells were then washed and carried through the NH$_4$Cl treatment.

After the NH$_4$Cl treatment the cells to be studied intact were resuspended in 0.85% saline, pelleted by centrifuging at 510 X g for ten minutes in a Lourdes Beta-Fuge Model A-2, and resuspended in the experimental media for a 30 minute incubation. The total final volume of cells plus incubation media was 12 ml. for use in an 8 mm NMR tube, and 2.5 ml for a 5 mm tube. The tubes require about 2.5 ml. and 0.5 ml. of packed cells respectively. The average number of packed cells/ml. is about 8 X 10^8 for EL-4 cells and 4 X 10^9 for spleen cells. After incubation, the cell suspensions were transferred to NMR tubes that had been packed tightly into centrifuge adapters with cotton wadding. The NMR tubes were then centrifuged in the Lourdes A-2 at 510 X g for 10 minutes for 5 mm tubes or 287 X g for 20 minutes for 8 mm tubes (to avoid breakage). The supernatant was then drawn off

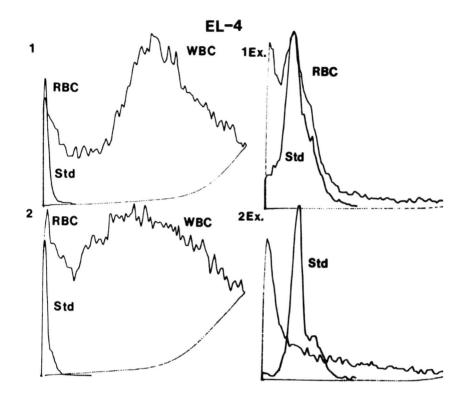

Fig. 2. Typical Coulter channelizer elect-
ronic cell volume distributions of an EL-4 tumor
cell (WBC) preparation. This illustrates the EL-4
tumor cell volume distributions before (1 and 1
expanded) and after (2 and 2 expanded) erythrocyte
(RBC) removal as compared to a peripheral blood
RBC standard. The vertical and horizontal scales
are number of cells and cell volume, respectively.
The volume of the EL-4 cells is about 590 cubic
microns.

with a pipet leaving the packed cells ready for NMR.

The membranes were prepared (see Fig. 3) by an extraction procedure originally developed by McCollester (8) and later modified by Warley and Cook (9). After NH_4Cl treatment the cells were pelleted by centrifuging at 500 X g for five minutes, then resuspended and washed twice in 10 X the packed cell volume (pcv) of harvesting solution (150 mM NaCl, 50 mM boric acid, 1.0 mM $CaCl_2$,

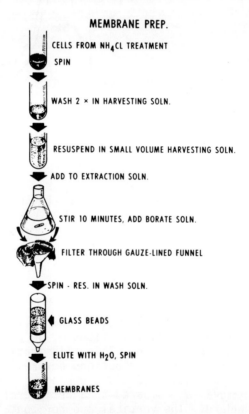

MEMBRANE PREP.

CELLS FROM NH_4CL TREATMENT

SPIN

WASH 2 × IN HARVESTING SOLN.

RESUSPEND IN SMALL VOLUME HARVESTING SOLN.

ADD TO EXTRACTION SOLN.

STIR 10 MINUTES, ADD BORATE SOLN.

FILTER THROUGH GAUZE-LINED FUNNEL

SPIN - RES. IN WASH SOLN.

GLASS BEADS

ELUTE WITH H_2O, SPIN

MEMBRANES

Fig. 3.   An outline of the EL-4 tumor and spleen white cell plasma membrane preparation procedure based on the method of Warley and Cook (9).

1.0 mM $MgCl_2$, pH 7.2), and repelleted. Next the cells were suspended in 2 X pcv of harvesting solution, and this suspension was added to an Erlenmeyer flask containing 200 X pcv of extraction solution (20 mM Na_2BO_3, 0.2 mM EDTA, pH 9.2). After stirring gently for ten minutes, 8 X pcv of 500 mM Na_2BO_3 (pH 9.6) was added, and the solution was filtered through gauze. The filtrate was then centrifuged at 2000 X g for 1.5 hours yielding a pellet which was subsequently resuspended in 25 X pcv of wash solution (2 mM Na_2BO_3, 1 mM EDTA) by vortexing. The resulting suspension was then applied to a column of 2 cm. i. d. containing 10 X pcv of glass beads (previously soaked in 0.1 M HCl and rinsed with distilled water until the effluent pH was 6.4). The membranes were eluted from the column with 15 X pcv of distilled water, and pelleted by centrifuging at 12,000 X g for 1 hour. The membranes were washed in deuterium oxide (D_2O) and pelleted by centrifugation three times before examination by NMR. Before NMR studies a dispersion of the membranes in D_2O was mildly sonicated by using two short bursts of about 30 seconds each at half the maximum output value with a Savant Insonator while the sample was packed in ice.

All NMR spectra were obtained using a Varian HA-100D-15 spectrometer operating at 100.0 MHz. in the HA mode. Signal averaging was employed for all spectra using a C-1024 computer. The water proton signal was used as the frequency lock signal in the intact cell and membrane spectra. Spectral calibrations are given in terms of parts per million (p.p.m.) upfield from the water signal in these spectra. The methyl signal from a reference compound sodium 2,2-dimethyl-2-silapentane-5- sulfonate (DSS) occurs at + 4.74 p.p.m. from the residual water proton peak in the membrane spectra and at + 4.65 p.p.m. in the intact cell spectra when DSS is added. The lipid extract spectra were calibrated in terms of p.p.m. downfield from the lock signal tetramethyl-silane (TMS).

For electron microscopic examination in the membrane pellet was fixed in 4% glutaraldehyde in 0.05 M sodium cacodylate buffer (pH 7.4). Post fixation was in 1% osmium tetroxide in 0.05 M sodium cacodylate buffer.

Dehydration was by 70%, 95% and 100% ethanol. The
sample was passed through three changes of Spur low
viscosity embedding medium, and flat embedded in this
medium at 70°c. overnight. Thin sections (gold) were
then prepared using a glass knife. The sections were
stained with uranyl acetate (saturated solution in 50%
ethanol) followed by lead citrate (10). Specimens
were examined using a Phillips 200 electron microscope.
This study showed that the preparation contained mainly
agranular membranes (Fig. 4) with no nuclear contamination, but some mitochondrial contamination.

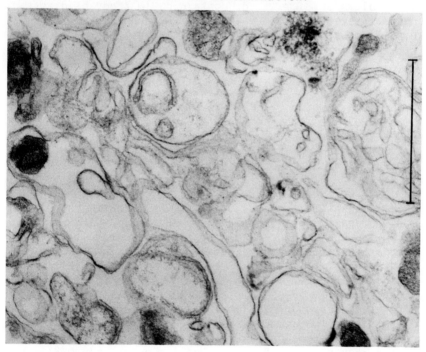

Fig. 4.   An electron micrograph showing the
types of materials present in the membrane preparation. The preparation is mainly agranular
membrane with no nuclear contamination, but with
some mitochondrial contamination. (The bar is 1
micron).

RESULTS AND DISCUSSION

The proton NMR spectra of the lipids in cells and membrane dispersions are actually more complicated than they may appear to be on a cursory examination. Only the signals from the most mobile of the lipid components are easily observed in high resolution spectra. Many other lipid components make subtle contributions to these spectra. In a model lipid system such as an egg lecithin dispersion it is believed (11) that only about 20% of the lipid chains are fairly mobile while the remainder have very restricted mobility. The mobile components make contributions to the spectra consisting of fairly sharp lines, while the less mobile fraction contributes much broader poorly resolved lines. In the case of sarcoplasmic reticulum membrane spectra for example, Davis and Inesi (4) have shown that about 80% of the lipid fatty acid chain protons give a very broad spectral contribution with a linewidth of about 500 Hz. About 20% of the lipids give rise to high resolution spectra with linewidths of about 20 Hz superimposed on the broad lines.

In the intact cell spectra the situation is more complex in that the very intense water peak is super-imposed on the spectra of other cellular components. In Fig. 5 the upfield portion of the spectra of intact EL-4 cells and normal mouse spleen white cells are shown. Easily observed here are high resolution peaks due to terminal CH_3-, lipid chain $-CH_2$-, $-CH_2CO$-, $-CH_2CH=C$, and $N^+(CH_3)_3$ protons. It is noted that the resonances in the EL-4 ascites tumor cell spectrum are much sharper and better resolved than those in the spleen cell spectrum. The reasons for these differences are not known at this time. In order to confirm these spectral assignments, samples of the tumor cells and the spleen cells were extracted with chloroform/methanol (2/1 vol.) to yield lipid extracts. The spectra of these extracts are shown in Fig. 6. Well resolved peaks are seen for terminal lipid chain and cholesterol CH_3-, $-CH_2$-, $-CH_2CH=C$, $-CH_2CO$-, $=CHCH_2CH=$, $-N^+(CH_3)_3$, $-OH$, and $-CH=C$ protons as well as the solvent CD_2HOD impurity. Resolution in these spectra is slightly limited due to the fact that the computer used in signal averaging only

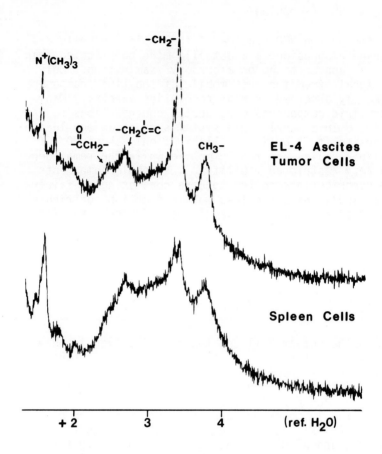

Fig. 5.   The 100 MHz proton NMR spectra of packed EL-4 cells and normal mouse spleen white cells.   The portion of the spectrum upfield from the water signal is shown.   A DSS methyl reference resonance would occur at + 4.65 p.p.m. on this scale. (70 scans, 8 mm o.d. tube).

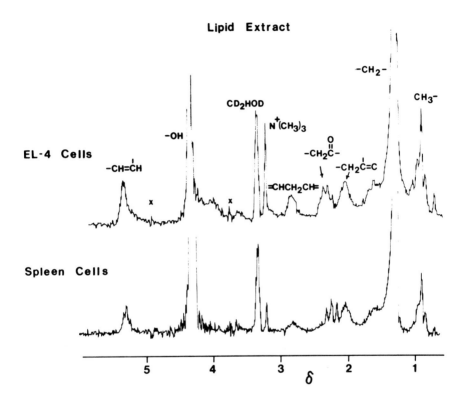

Fig. 6. The 100 MHz proton NMR spectra of lipid extracts of EL-4 cells and normal mouse spleen white cells in deuterated chloroform/ methanol (2/1, vol.). (36 scans, ref. TMS).

has 1024 channels and the instrument sweep width is 1000 Hz. The spectral assignments are consistent with those previously reported in the literature. The significance of the minor differences in the spectra of these extracts has as yet not been fully explored. It is apparent that the spectra in Fig. 5 show a strong resemblance to the upfield portion of the spectra in Fig. 6 with the exception that all lines are somewhat broadened in the former spectra, especially in the case of the spleen cells.

If the lipid peaks in Fig. 5 contain a contribution from plasma membrane lipids, the peak intensities should show variation with changes in the composition of the incubation medium as reported by Cerbón. In Fig. 7 the results of such a set of experiments is shown. These cells were run in 5 mm tubes and were spun at a higher centrifugal force than those in Fig. 5 causing some line broadening, but the effects are still apparent. Changing the incubation medium from isotonic saline to either hypotonic saline or to a $CaCl_2$ solution causes an increase in the intensity of the $-CH_2-$ proton resonances. However, this effect is much smaller than that observed by Cerbón.

Any contributions to the spectra that arise from plasma membrane lipids may be affected by phenomena which are known to involve the cell surface components. Previous workers (12) have found that concanavillin A (Con A) can be used to coat EL-4 ascites tumor cells. Consequently it was thought that such a treatment might be used as a probe to further determine if plasma membrane lipids are visible in the NMR spectra of whole cells. In Fig. 8 the effect of incubation of 5×10^9 cells in 12.5 ml of saline containing 54 mg Con A at 37°c. for 30 minutes is shown. A general broadening effect is seen in the spectra of the Con A treated EL-4 cells as compared to the untreated cells. In fact there appears to be a differential broadening effect on the $-CH_2-$ resonances as compared to the $-N^+(CH_3)_3$ resonances. At least three factors can cause line broadening in the Con A treated sample: 1) decreased mobility of the lipid chains, 2) paramagnetic broadening due to the presence of Mn^{++} in the Con A, and 3) increased sample inhomogeneity effects due to cell agglutination. The effect of Mn^{++} on the

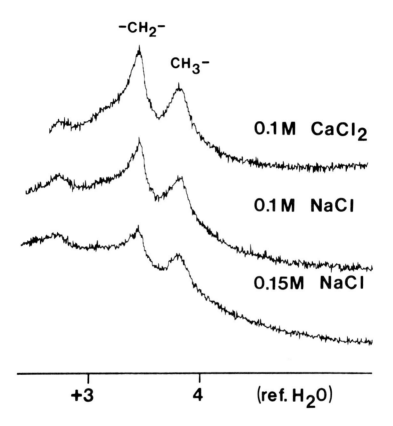

Fig. 7. The upfield portions of the 100 MHz proton NMR spectra of packed EL-4 cells incubated with 0.1 m $CaCl_2$, 0.1 M NaCl and 0.15 M NaCl for 30 min. prior to centrifugation. (25 scans, 5 mm o.d. tubes).

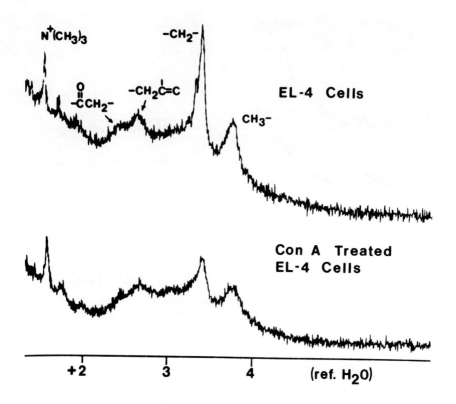

Fig. 8.   The upfield protions of the 100
MHz proton NMR spectra of packed EL-4 cells with
and without Con A treatment (70 scans, 8 mm o.d.
tubes).

spectrum was investigated by incubating the cells with several concentrations of $MnCl_2$ in saline. As the concentration of Mn^{++} increases, the water linewidth increases dramatically while the lipid peaks remain relatively unchanged until the water signal completely obscures the lipid signals. Since this behavior is completely different from that observed upon addition of Con A to the cells, paramagnetic broadening due to Mn^{++} is probably not the cause of line broadening in the case of the Con A treated cells. Although increased inhomogeneity effects are a possibility, no macroscopic clumps were observed in the Con A treated samples. The linewidths appear to be differentially broadened, i.e., the $-CH_2-$ peak appears to be broadened more than the $N^+(CH_3)_3$ peak. This indicates that the line broadening mechanism is probably not one which involves an increase in sample magnetic inhomogeneity. Thus it appears that restricted mobility of lipid chains is the likely cause of the line broadening.

Although the intact cell studies are very interesting, they might be considered a rather indirect means of studying plasma membranes. In addition, those spectra may contain some contributions from other cellular components. Consequently, plasma membranes were prepared for study from both EL-4 and normal spleen white cells. Initially a density gradient preparation technique (13) was used, however agglutination of membrane vesicles severely limited the yields. Consequently the extraction procedure of Warley and Cook (9) was used for this study. A spectrum of the EL-4 membranes dispersed in deuterium oxide by vortexing and mild sonication is shown in Fig. 9. Clearly visible are the peaks due to the terminal CH_3-, lipid chain $-CH_2-$, and $N^+(CH_3)_3$ protons. It is noted that this spectrum shows a striking resemblance to that of the intact EL-4 cells with the exception that the lines are slightly broader here. In the case of the spleen cell membranes, spectra could not be obtained using such mild treatment. The latter membranes aggregated and precipitated out of the dispersion too quickly to obtain a time averaged NMR spectrum.

Lee, Birdsall, and Metcalfe (14) have made a detailed examination of the NMR linewidths of lipid chain

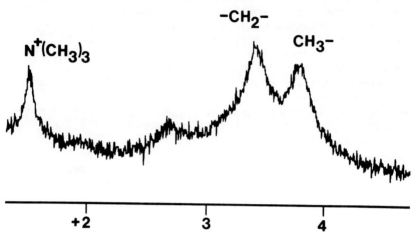

Fig. 9.   The upfield portion of the 100
MHz proton NMR spectrum of EL-4 ascites tumor
plasma membranes dispersed in deuterium oxide.
A DSS methyl reference resonance would occur at
+ 4.74 p.p.m. on this scale. (250 scans, 12 mm
tube).

methylene protons. Their work indicates that the proton
transverse relaxation is due primarily to dipolar inter-
actions and that the dominant relaxation mechanism arises
from translational self-diffusion of the lipid chains.
Charvolin and Rigny (15) have reached similar conclusions
from a pulsed NMR study of a potassium laurate system.
In both of these studies estimates of the self-diffusion
coefficients of the lipid chains were made using the NMR
data.   The former treatment which is based on the works
of Resing and Torrey (16) and of Kruger (17) is readily
applicable to the continuous wave studies reported here.
In the former treatment, the contribution to the linewidth that is due to dipolar relaxation is given as a
function of two variables. By making reasonable assump-
tions about the value of one of the variables (based on
experimental evidence from other systems), Lee et al.,
were able to generate a plot of the dipolar linewidth

as a function of the self-diffusion coefficient (D). Since the dipolar linewidth is always less than or equal to the experimental linewidth, such a plot allows an estimate of the lower limit of D to be made from the -CH$_2$- proton linewidth. The plot generated by Lee et al. was used to estimate the lower limits for D for the mobile lipid components in intact cell and membrane preparations used in this study (see Table 1).

Table 1.

Lipid Chain Methyene Proton Signals

Sample	Est. Linewidth(Hz)	Lower Limit of D x 10^9(cm^2/sec)
Intact EL-4	14	~6.5
Con A treated EL-4	20-30	3-4.5
EL-4 membrane	56	1.5
Extracted Lipids in CD$_3$OD/CDCl$_3$	6	15
Literature (14)		
Sarcoplasmic reticulum membrane, 8°	15	6
Extracted Lipid, 31°	22	4
Electroplax membrane	<75	1

It is interesting that the lower limit estimate for D is less for the Con A treated cells than for the untreated EL-4 cells. This could reflect slower diffusion of the lipid chains in the Con A treated sample. The EL-4 membranes show a lower limit for D which is less than that found for the intact cells. At present it is

269

not known whether these findings reflect accurately
differences in D or whether other line-broadening effects
are significant. As expected, the lipids studied here
appear to be the most mobile in the extracts solubilized
in chloroform-methanol mixtures. A comparison of the
values for the lower limit of D found in this study
with those obtained by Lee et al. shows that they are
all in the same general range. These values also agree
with the average diffusion coefficient estimated by
Charvolin and Rigny for potassium laurate chains (1.5 X
10^{-9} cm^2/sec.).

CONCLUSIONS

Intact EL-4 cells and normal mouse spleen cells have
NMR patterns that appear to arise from cellular lipids.
The spectra from the intact EL-4 cells resemble the
spectra of isolated plasma membranes. In addition, the
NMR patterns of the intact EL-4 cells show variations
with changes in the osmolarity and with the presence
of divalent ions in the incubation medium. These signals
also show changes upon the addition of Con A, a substance
known to interact with cell surface sites. The mobilities
of the lipids giving rise to these intact cell signals
appear to be in the same range as those observed for other
membrane lipids. Consequently, it appears that at least
part of the lipid signals observed with the intact cells
are probably due to plasma membrane lipids. These
studies indicate that information concerning membrane
structure and properties might be obtained from NMR
studies of intact tumor cells as well as from studies
of the isolated membranes.

ACKNOWLEDGEMENTS

Dr. D. Smith and Ms. M. Hart of the PCRI staff are
gratefully acknowledged for performing the electron
microscopy. This work was supported in part by N.I.H
Grant No. CA-13056-02 from the National Cancer Institute.
The N.I.H. (Grant No. AM-13966) and the Florida Division
of the American Cancer Society are gratefully acknowledged
for past contributions toward the purchase of the NMR
spectrometer.

REFERENCES

1. D. Chapman and V.B. Kamat, in: Regulatory Functions of Biological Membranes, ed. J. Jarnfelt (Elsevier, New York, 1968) p. 99.

2. S.Joffe and R.E. Block, Brain Res. 46 (1972) 381.

3. R.E. Block, A.H. Brady, and S. Joffe, Biochem. Biophys. Res. Commun. 54 (1973) 1595.

4. D.G. Davis and G. Inesi, Biochim. Biophys. Acta 241 (1971) 1.

5. J. Cerbon, Biochim. Biophys. Acta 102 (1965) 499.

6. G.F. Schwartz, Exp. Med. Surg. 29 (1971) 1.

7. P.A. Gorer, Brit. J. Cancer 4 (1950) 372.

8. D.L. McCollester, Cancer Research 30 (1970) 2832.

9. A. Warley and G.M.W. Cook, Biochim. Biophys. Acta 323 (1973) 55.

10. E.S. Reynolds, J. Cell Biol. 17 (1963) 208.

11. A.F. Horwitz, W.J. Horsley, and M.P. Klein, Proc. Nat. Acad. Sci. U.S.A. 69 (1972) 590.

12. W.J. Martin, E. Esber, and J.R. Wunderlich, Fed. Proc. 32 (1973) 173.

13. A.M. Woodin and A.A. Wieneke, Biochem. J. 99 (1966) 479.

14. A.G. Lee, N.J.M. Birdsall, and J.C. Metcalfe, Biochemistry 12 (1973) 1650.

15. J. Charvolin and P. Rigny, J. Magn. Resonance 4 (1971) 40.

16. H.A. Resing and H.C. Torrey, Phys. Rev. 131 (1963) 1102.

17. G.J. Kruger, Z. Naturforsch 24A (1969) 560.

DISCUSSION

H.J. Heiniger, Jackson Laboratory: In your slide where you depicted the lipid extract from the EL-4 cells and the lymphocytes, I thought I saw that the peak of the cholesterol was much larger in your EL-4 cells than in the normal lymphocytes. Is this correct? It interests me because of our recent findings on cholesterol synthesis in leukemic mouse cells (Cancer Research 33, 2774-2778, 1973).

R.E. Block, Papanicolaou Cancer Research Institute: It is apparently much larger. We don't know if this is due to an inefficient extraction procedure or if it is in fact indicating a larger amount of cholesterol in the EL-4.

J. Jaroszewski, Naval Medical Research Institute: There is an evidence coming from our laboratory that ammonium chloride treatment inflicts an injury to T lymphocytes, both in mice and in humans. Do you have any proof that your ammonium chloride treatment didn't cause any artifacts?

R.E. Block: I know exactly what you're talking about. We've worried about this quite a bit. First of all, the viabilities that we get after ammonium chloride treatment are greater than 90%. In other words, we're losing all the dead cells essentially. The second criterion is: if you take the ammonium chloride treated tumor cells and inject them into mice, you get tumors. The tumors that arise take about 2 days longer than with the untreated cells, so this would indicate that there might be some slight damage but we don't know exactly the extent of it.

W. Korytnyk, Roswell Park Memorial Institute: There have been several reports in the literature according to which the water relaxation times of cancer cells are significantly longer than those of normal cells. Have you been able to confirm these observations?

   R.E. Block: We've confirmed it on solid tissues (for examples see: R.E. Block, (Fed. Eur. Bioch. Soc.) FEBS Lett. 34 (1973) 109; R.E. Block and G.P. Maxwell, J. Magn. Resonance 14, (1974) in press.) We have not confirmed it on this system.

ALTERATIONS OF COMPLEX LIPID METABOLISM IN TUMORIGENIC DNA AND RNA VIRUS-TRANSFORMED CELLS

ROSCOE O. BRADY and PETER H. FISHMAN
Developmental and Metabolic Neurology Branch
National Institute of Neurological Diseases and Stroke
National Institutes of Health, Bethesda, Maryland 20014

Abstract: Mouse cell lines which exhibit contact-inhibi-
tion of growth in culture contain a homologous series
of gangliosides ranging in size from monosialosyl-
lactosylceramide to disialosyltetrahexosylceramide.
The size of the oligosaccharide chains in these
membrane-associated glycolipids is reduced when cells
are transformed with tumorigenic DNA and RNA viruses.
These alterations in ganglioside pattern are due to
specific blocks in the biosynthesis of gangliosides
in the transformed cells.

INTRODUCTION

Gangliosides comprise a group of acidic glycolipids
which are primarily localized in membranous elements of
mammalian cells. Normal mouse cell lines contain a
family of these substances whose structures are indicated
in Fig. 1. Since these lipids are highly concentrated in
plasma cell membranes, we reasoned that an examination of
the composition of these materials in control and tumorigenic virus-transformed cells might provide insight into
biochemical alterations which attend neoplastic transformations. We discovered that the pattern of gangliosides
is dramatically changed as a consequence of virus transformation and we have pinpointed the metabolic alterations
which are responsible for these changes.

275

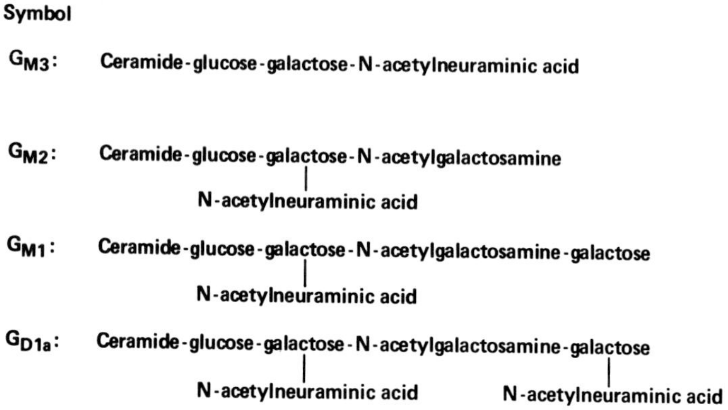

Symbol

G_{M3}: Ceramide-glucose-galactose-N-acetylneuraminic acid

G_{M2}: Ceramide-glucose-galactose-N-acetylgalactosamine
                                                 |
                           N-acetylneuraminic acid

G_{M1}: Ceramide-glucose-galactose-N-acetylgalactosamine-galactose
                                                 |
                           N-acetylneuraminic acid

G_{D1a}: Ceramide-glucose-galactose-N-acetylgalactosamine-galactose
                                                 | |
                           N-acetylneuraminic acid   N-acetylneuraminic acid

Fig. 1.   Gangliosides of normal mouse cell lines.

EXPERIMENTAL

Cells and Cell Culture

We have generally employed the 3 principal mouse strains AL/N, Balb/c and Swiss mouse lines which are in wide usage throughout the world. The derivative lines we investigated were transformed with the tumorigenic DNA viruses Simian virus 40 (SV40), polyoma virus (Py), or the Moloney isolate of murine sarcoma virus (MSV) and the Kirsten strain of murine sarcoma virus (KiMSV) which are RNA viruses. We also examined the effect of non-transforming "helper" viruses such as murine leukemia virus. The AL/N cell lines were grown in Eagle's medium. Dulbecco's modification of Eagle's medium supplemented with 10% fetal calf serum was used for the other cell lines. The cells were harvested by mechanical scraping, brief trypsinization, or with 0.5% EDTA. In several experiments, labeled ganglioside precursors such as N-acetyl-[^{3}H]-mannosamine or $\underline{D}$-glucosamine-^{14}C were added to the incubation medium.

Isolation of Gangliosides and Assay of Glycosyltransferases

Gangliosides were extracted from washed packed cells by homogenization in 20 volumes of a solution of chloroform-methanol (2:1, v/v) as previously described (1). The gangliosides were separated by thin-layer chromatography and quantitated by chromogenic or densitometric procedures (2). Gangliosides were also quantified by gas-liquid chromatographic analysis of appropriate derivatives of the sugar components (3). The incorporation of label into gangliosides was determined with a chromatogram scanning device (2).

Enzyme assays were generally performed by suspending the washed packed cells in 9 volumes of 0.25 $\underline{M}$ sucrose solution with 0.1% 2-mercaptoethanol. The suspension was frozen and thawed 4 times to disrupt the cells (4). The biosynthesis of gangliosides occurs by the step-wise addition of monosaccharides from sugar nucleotide donors to the growing glycolipid acceptor via a series of reactions catalyzed by specific glycosyltransferases (Fig. 2). The assay mixtures contained the glycolipid acceptor, nucleotide donor, detergent and Mn^{++} where required, and sodium cacodylate buffer at the appropriate pH for the various reactions (4-6). The reactions were stopped by the addition of 20 volumes of a solution of $CHCl_3$-MeOH, and the products were separated from the labeled substrates by gel filtration as previously described (4).

RESULTS AND DISCUSSION

Distribution of Gangliosides in Normal and Virally Transformed Cells

There is a striking difference in the pattern of gangliosides in SV40 or Py virus-transformed mouse cells compared with normal or spontaneously transformed cells (1). This change is characterized by the absence of all of the ganglioside homologs larger than G_{M3}. A typical

277

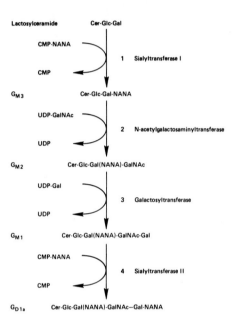

Fig. 2. Biosynthetic steps in the formation of gangliosides

thin-layer chromatogram of gangliosides in contact-inhibited and DNA virus-transformed Swiss mouse cells is shown in Fig. 3. A similar alteration of the ganglioside pattern occurs in DNA virus-transformed AL/N (Table 1) and Balb/c cells (7). The same change in ganglioside composition occurred when Swiss mouse cells were transformed with the Moloney isolate of MSV (8).

A slightly different alteration in the ganglioside pattern was found when Balb/c 3T3 cells were transformed with KiMSV. The transformed cells contained G_{M2} in addi-

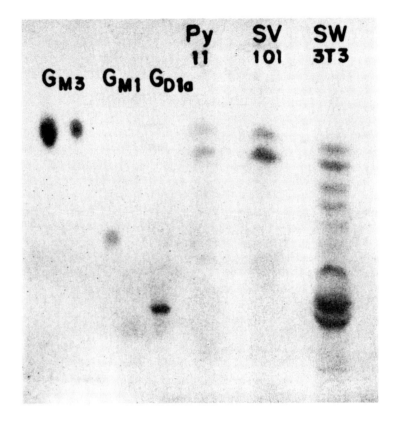

Fig. 3. Ganglioside patterns in normal (3T3), SV40, and Py virus-transformed Swiss mouse cells.

tion to G_{M3} which is the only ganglioside in the SV40, Py, and MSV transformed cells (6). The pattern and labelling of gangliosides in KiMSV-transformed Balb/c cells grown in the presence of $\underline{D}$-glucosamine-^{14}C are shown in Fig. 4.

Enzyme Studies
The alteration in ganglioside distribution could conceivably be due to either increased catabolism or decreased synthesis of the higher homologs. The major ganglioside in normal mouse cells is G_{D1a} and in DNA virus-transformed cells is G_{M3}. Both of these lipids have a

279

TABLE 1

Distribution of gangliosides in normal (N AL/N), SV40, and
Py virus-transformed derivative lines

| Cell type | Ganglioside | | | | |
	G_{D1a}	G_{M1}	G_{M2}	G_{M3}	Total
	nanomoles/mg of protein				
N AL/N	1.8	1.5	0.8	0.6	4.7
SV40 AL/N	0.16	0.22	0.1	1.9	2.4
Py AL/N	0.1	0.15	0.2	1.8	2.3

terminal molecule of sialic acid and their catabolism is
initiated through the activity of a neuraminidase on the
respective compounds (9). We investigated these initial
hydrolytic reactions in contact-inhibited and DNA virus-
transformed cells and found that the activity of these
catabolic enzymes was essentially the same in the two
types of cells (5). We then undertook an investigation
of the specific reactions involved in the biosynthesis of
gangliosides. Since G_{M3} is present in the DNA virus-
transformed cell lines but more complex homologs are
virtually absent, the activity of the aminosugar transferase involved in the synthesis of G_{M2} from G_{M3} (Fig. 2,
Reaction 2) was examined. This enzyme is present in homogenates of contact-inhibited and spontaneously transformed
mouse cell lines. The activity of the enzyme is drasti-
cally reduced in SV40 and Py virus-transformed cells and
cells transformed by the Moloney isolate of MSV (Table 2).

The altered pattern of gangliosides in the KiMSV transformed Balb/c cells suggested that the activity of the
galactosyltransferase which catalyzes the conversion of
G_{M2} to G_{M1} (Fig. 2, Reaction 3) was impaired in these
cells. Our investigations indicated that this was the
metabolic block in ganglioside synthesis in the KiMSV

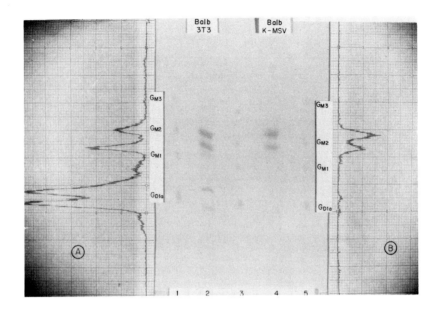

Fig. 4. Gangliosides and labelling patterns of normal
Balb/c 3T3 and KiMSV-transformed Balb/c cells grown
in the presence of $\underline{\underline{D}}$-glucosamine-^{14}C.

transformed cells (Table 3).

Effect of Growth and Culture Conditions on Ganglioside Metabolism

Normal cells in culture will cease dividing when they
come into contact with one another. Transformed cells
continue to grow and divide after making contact and will
reach a high saturation density in culture. No effect
was observed on the ganglioside content of the cells when
the density was varied by changing the length of time in
culture. In addition, the possible influence of cell
density on the ganglioside synthesizing enzymes was carefully explored with Swiss 3T3 cells. There was no significant change in the activities of the four glycosyltransferases listed in Fig. 2 over a ten-fold range in

TABLE 2

UDP-N-acetylgalactosamine: G_{M3}-N-acetylgalactosaminyltransferase activity in mouse cell lines

Cell line	Growth in culture	Enzyme activity
		(percent of controls)
N AL/N	Contact-inhibited	100
SV40 AL/N	High cell density	16
Py AL/N	High cell density	14
Swiss 3T3	Contact-inhibited	100
Swiss SV40	High cell density	13
Swiss Py	High cell density	17
Swiss MSV	High cell density	20

Data calculated from References 4 and 8.

Table 3

Glycosyltransferase activities in Balb/c 3T3 and KiMSV-transformed Balb/c 3T3 cells

Cell line	N-acetylgalactosaminyl-transferase	Galactosyltransferase	
	Whole homogenate	Whole homogenate	Washed particles
	nanomoles per mg of protein per hr		
Balb/c 3T3	2.51	0.25	0.58
KBalb/c	2.58	<0.015	<0.015

Summary of data from Ref. 6.

cell density (4).

Lytic Infection of Cells

Mouse cells are permissive for Py virus which infects these cells with production of numerous virus particles and only rarely are the cells transformed (10). Both AL/N and Swiss 3T3 cells were infected with a high multiplicity of Py virus particles. The cells underwent lysis at 4-7 days indicating successful lytic infection. There was no effect on the activity of the N-acetylgalactosaminyltransferase in the infected cells (11). In addition, there was no change in the activity of this enzyme when Swiss 3T3 cells were infected with Moloney leukemia virus (8) or change in ganglioside pattern when Balb/c 3T3 cells were infected with Rauscher leukemia virus. These results indicate that the reduced aminosugar transferase activity in virally transformed cells is specifically associated with some transforming function of these viruses.

Phenotypic Reversion of Growth Properties and Altered Ganglioside Metabolism

Since the change in ganglioside biosynthesis appears to be related to transformation, the question arises whether the presence of an integrated viral genome is sufficient to produce this change. Phenotypic "flat revertant" cloned lines derived from SV40 and Py virus-transformed Swiss 3T3 cells (12) were examined for ganglioside composition. In the "flat revertant" SV40 line which is now contact-inhibited, the ganglioside pattern was similar to the normal contact-inhibited Swiss 3T3 cell line and is in stark contrast to the ganglioside pattern in the non-contact-inhibited SV40 transformed cells (Table 4). The flat revertant line derived from Py virus-transformed cells showed phenotypic and genotypic heterogeneity (13). The ganglioside pattern was only partially restored in these cells.

The levels of N-acetylgalactosaminyl transferase activity in these cells accurately reflects the ganglioside patterns. It is fully restored in the "flat" SV40 and partially restored in the "flat" Py revertant cell line (11). A similar restoration of aminosugar transferase activity was observed in a "flat" clonal line selected out from SV40 transformed Balb/c mouse cells by dependence on

283

TABLE 4

Distribution of gangliosides in Swiss 3T3, SV40, and Py virus-transformed derivative lines and in flat sublines derived from the virus-transformed lines

Cell line	Ganglioside				
	G_{D1a}	G_{M1}	G_{M2}	G_{M3}	Total
	nanomoles/mg of protein				
Swiss 3T3	1.8	1.4	1.3	3.3	7.8
SV40	0.05	0.1	0.05	3.5	3.7
Py	0.1	0.2	0.05	3.2	3.5
F1 SV40	2.6	0.8	1.4	2.8	7.7
F1 Py	0.93	0.2	0.4	3.9	5.4

From Ref. 11

a serum growth factor (14).

The results indicate that the altered ganglioside metabolism as manifested by the activity of the N-acetylgalactosaminyltransferase is coordinately linked to the phenotypic growth properties of these virally transformed mouse cells. Thus, a biochemical expression of transformation appears to be coupled to the morphological expression of transformation. The tumor virus is integrated into the host cell DNA in these "flat revertant" cells, T-antigen is produced which indicates expression of some viral properties, and in the case of SV40, virus can be rescued from these cells. It therefore appears that the expression of certain viral functions can be modulated by the host cell. Thus, integration of the viral genome into host cell DNA is not sufficient for the occurrence of an altered ganglioside metabolism. However, when the restoration of the ganglioside pattern and synthesis was compared with the karyotype of the various cell lines, a potentially significant correlation seems to appear. The "flat revertant" SV40 transformed cells had an increased number of chromosomes above the subtetraploid level seen in the parent 3T3 and SV40 transformant. The partially reverted Py virus-transformed cells were phenotypically heterogeneous with morphological features intermediate between the large, flattened contact-inhibited parent cells and the smaller, rounded virus-transformed cells. The ganglioside pattern and the aminosugar transferase activity were also intermediate between that in the parent and transformed cells. The partially reverted Py transformant exhibited some of the hyperploidy seen in the SV40 flat revertant, but there was a significant decrease from the subtetraploid number of chromosomes in a large percentage of these cells (13). Accordingly, we are tempted to suggest that a correlation exists between the number of chromosomes and the activity of the N-acetylgalactosaminyltransferase in the flat revertant cells.

Search for a Transmissible Repressor

Because G_{M3}:UDP-N-acetylgalactosaminyltransferase activity was decreased in cells transformed with tumorigenic DNA viruses, it is conceivable that a common diffusible repressor substance might be produced by cells transformed by these viruses. In order to investigate this possibility contact-inhibited and virus-transformed cells were grown under a common medium but separated from each other by a ridge in the center of the culture flask. The cells were harvested separately and the activity of the aminosugar transferase was determined in each of the two types of cells. There was no evidence of diffusion of an inhibitory factor from the virus-transformed cells to the contact-inhibited normal cells (11). There also was no indication of correction of diminished activity of the aminosugar transferase in the transformed cells by a "metabolic cooperativity factor" from the control cells.

The possibility exists that a non-diffusible repressor might be produced in the transformed cell which can pass from cell to cell if they are sufficiently close to each other. In order to examine this aspect, control and virus-transformed cells were grown in an intimate admixture. The distribution of the two types of cells at harvest was

285

determined by immunological identification of the transformed cells. The activity of the aminosugar transferase
was then assayed in a homogenate of the mixed cells. There
was 36% less activity of this enzyme in such homogenates
than the value calculated on the basis of the estimated
number of the two types of cells in the culture (11). It
is very difficult to decide whether this decrease is
significant or can be attributed to flaws in the design
and execution of this experiment. However, when the two
types of cells were grown separately, harvested, and then
homogenized together, the value obtained on assay for
aminosugar transferase was almost exactly that predicted
from that observed in the respective cells assayed separately (5,11). These observations seem to indicate clearly
that there was no accumulation of an inhibitor of the
aminosugar transferase in the virus-transformed cells.

*Generality of the Phenomenon of Impaired Ganglioside
Synthesis in Virus Transformation of Cells*

We have observed a marked decrease in G_{M3}:UDP-N-acetyl-
galactosaminyltransferase activity in 24 out of 26 individually transformed mouse cell line with tumorigenic DNA
viruses which were available for our examination (14-16).
The pattern of gangliosides was consistently altered in
the 24 lines in keeping with the block of this biosynthetic
step in ganglioside formation. One of the exceptions
which we analyzed was an SV40 transformed mouse cell line
selected for resistance to 5-bromo-2-deoxyuridine (17).
The second exception was a temperature-sensitive SV40
transformed Swiss 3T3 cell line. The latter line is unusual in that the temperature-sensitive mutation is host-
cell related since wild type virus can be rescued from
these cells (18). Alteration of ganglioside composition
similar to that observed by us in mouse cell lines has
also been reported by Sheinin and co-workers (19), Nigam
et al. in hamster lines (20), and by Wiblin and Macpherson
in a very interesting experiment in which SV40 transformed
baby hamster kidney cells were hybridized with 3T3 mouse
cells (21). However, in addition to the two exceptions
which we observed, reports of three other exceptions to
this phenomenon have appeared (22,23).

The ganglioside changes observed in tumorigenic RNA
virus-transformed mouse cells appear to be more complex.

286

Following mass infection and transformation of Swiss and Balb/c 3T3 cells with the Moloney isolate of MSV, there is a dramatic decrease in aminosugar transferase activity in these cells (8). The same enzyme change was observed in an established clonal line of Balb/c 3T3 cells which, while leukemia virus negative, do produce type C particles (24). However, a clonal line of Balb/c 3T3 cells transformed by the Kirsten isolate of MSV has normal levels of aminosugar transferase activity but an absence of G_{M2}:UDP-galactosyltransferase activity (6). The latter transformed cell line does not produce any virus particles (25). However, the ganglioside pattern of a non-producer clone of Balb/c 3T3 cells transformed by another stock of Moloney sarcoma virus (25) showed an accumulation of G_{M2}, but also exhibited reduced amount of G_{D1a}. The two stocks of Moloney sarcoma virus appear to be different as leukemia virus negative clones transformed by the first stock do produce type C particles whereas clones transformed by the other stock are non-producers. Until these difference amongst the various isolates of murine sarcoma viruses can be clarified, the relationship between transformation by these viruses and the observed alterations in ganglioside metabolism cannot be fully delineated.

Molecular Basis of Altered Ganglioside Metabolism in Virus-Transformed Cells

Our investigations indicate that the tumorigenic virus genome must be inserted into the host cell DNA in order to effect the changes in ganglioside pattern and synthesis which we have observed. We now consider how the tumorigenic virus genome causes the decrease in the activity of the aminosugar transferase which occurs with tumorigenic DNA viruses and the Moloney isolate of MSV and the galactosyltransferase in cells transformed with KiMSV. The various possibilities include modification of enzymatic activity at the level of DNA transcription, at the level of messenger RNA translation, reduction of enzymatic activity by an inhibitor, or allosteric modification of the catalytic properties of these glycosyltransferases. Our knowledge of regulation of gene expression in mammalian cells is minute compared with our understanding of bacterial systems. However, several intelligent speculations can be made based on the data available.

A. The viral DNA may integrate into host cell chromosomes at the locus of the cistron coding for the affected
glycosyltransferase. Insertion of this non-host DNA may
interfere with transcription of this gene or cause a frame-
shift mutation resulting in the production of an inactive
or only partially active enzyme. Such an insertion of a
tumorigenic virus could account for the decreased activity
of the glycosyltransferases as well as the occasional non-
obligatoriness of the metabolic alteration. There are
several lines of evidence which argue against this model.
1. Viral DNA is also integrated during productive infection
of cells (27,28) which does not affect ganglioside metabolism in mouse cells. However, it is possible that the
integration of virus occurs at a site during such a lytic
infection which does not result in tumorigenic transformation of the cell and the attendant changes in ganglioside
metabolism. 2. Flat revertant cell lines also contain
integrated viral genomes which can express at least one
viral function, tumor antigen production, but still have
phenotypic properties of the parent contact-inhibited
cells and a normal complement of gangliosides. It should
be remembered that the particular flat-revertant cells
in which these effects occurred exhibited hyperploidy and
it is possible that an unaffected host gene coded for the
active aminosugar transferase in these cells.

In spite of these potential objections, the integration
site model is attractive for several reasons. 1. It is
sufficiently flexible so that we can understand why there
are exceptions to the general phenomenon of altered ganglioside metabolism in tumorigenic virus-transformed cells.
Studies with hybrid cells indicate that the viral genome
can be associated with more than one chromosome, presumably
in a random fashion (29,30). Thus, integration of the
viral genome into one particular host chromosome would be
required for an alteration of ganglioside metabolism. 2.
This model is compatible with the observation that
different strains of virus bring about different blocks in
the biosynthesis of gangliosides since viral integration
may have occurred at different gene loci. 3. It could
explain the occasionally observed alteration in the activity of more than one glycosyltransferase involved in
ganglioside synthesis. This situation is analogous to the
phenomenon of polarity in bacteria where a mutation in one

gene of a polycistron alters the translation of subsequent genes.

B. The induction and repression of enzyme synthesis in eukaryotic cells can occur at the level of messenger RNA. Thus, SV40, Py virus, and MSV could contain the genetic information for a common repressor molecule which inter- feres with the synthesis of the aminosugar transferase. The two DNA viruses can code for 5 to 10 polypeptides and the potential coding capacity of the larger quantity of genetic material in the tumorigenic RNA viruses is exten- sive. However, this proposal does not provide a ready explanation for the return of higher ganglioside synthesis in the flat revertant cell lines. If the model were analogous to the condition in bacterial systems, one would anticipate that the hypothetical repressor would be dominant. On the other hand, the existence of the flat revertants strongly suggests that host cell factors are involved in the expression of the transformed phenotype. Little is known about the regulation of glycolipid syn- thesis, but studies in synchronized cell populations indicate that cellular control mechanisms do exist since there are marked fluctuations in the activity of these enzymes throughout the cell cycle. It is conceivable that a viral gene product could interfere with the normal regulation and biosynthesis of these compounds. This mechanism would also explain the elevated levels of glycosyltransferases other than the depressed reaction since an impairment of negative feed-back control might result in continual expression of these enzyme activities.

Relationship between Altered Ganglioside Metabolism and Tumorigenicity

At this point we should like to offer some specula- tions concerning the potential significance of the altera- tions in ganglioside composition and metabolism to tumori- genic virus transformation. Such changes may be relevant only if they explain the altered social behavior of trans- formed cells in culture and in vivo. Tumorigenic virus- transformed cells in general exhibit a loss of growth control and certain structural and immunological changes on the cell surface (31). We are therefore concerned with the transmission of membrane-mediated information -- both externally and internally and how this transmission has been altered by virus transformation. If we conceptualize the plasma cell membrane as a fluid mosaic (32), then the carbohydrate chains of glycolipids and glycoproteins would be conceived as polar entities floating above a hydrophobic environment. The informational potential of these groups is tremendous and most likely is involved in cell-cell recognition phenomena (33,34). Structural and topographical variation may well influence behavior involving cell-cell recognition and adhesiveness, contact inhibition of growth, surface antigens, agglutination sites, substratum and serum factor requirements, and neoplastic transformation. The role of gangliosides in any or all of these phenomena is by no means clear at this moment. It should be remembered that we have stressed from the beginning of our investigations in this field that the pattern and synthesis of gangliosides in cells which have apparently undergone spontaneous transformation in vitro to the tumorigenic state may be normal as far as we can tell at this time (1). What we are concerned with here are the alterations of ganglioside composition and synthesis which appear to be a direct consequence of transformation of cells with oncogenic viruses. Exposure of cells to non-transforming viruses even at a very high multiplicity of infection does not produce these changes in ganglioside metabolism. Therefore we postulate that the changes in gangliosides are direct consequences of tumorigenic virus transformation and we are obligated to consider what role if any is played by gangliosides in mediating the behavior of cells.

Gangliosides may interact directly in such phenomena or indirectly by masking or unmasking other informational groups. Plasma membranes are enriched in gangliosides (35, 36), and the altered ganglioside pattern of virus-transformed cells is also reflected in their plasma membranes (19). One example of ganglioside involvement in the external flow of membrane information is the finding that ganglioside G_{M1} is the specific receptor for cholera toxin (37). Interaction of the toxin with the G_{M1} receptor results in a stimulation of adenyl cyclase and an increase in intracellular cyclic AMP levels. Transformed cells lacking G_{M1} are not as responsive to cholera toxin as normal cells (38). We would like to speculate that gangliosides act as receptors for other external factors found in serum or excreted from cells in culture. The absence of these receptors on the surfaces of transformed cells could explain their lack of response to such factors. One example is the ability of virally transformed cells to grow in serum factor-free media (39).

The internal transmission of membrane-mediated information between the plasma membrane and cell nucleus is also important to the regulation of growth. The cell surface is not isolated from the nucleus as there is a vast intracellular network of membranous structures which contains glycolipids, glycoproteins, and glycosyltransferases. Evidence is now accumulating that the metabolism and composition of complex carbohydrates change during the cell cycle. Glycolipids (40) and gangliosides (41) appear to be synthesized and incorporated into cell membranes during cell division. Thus, if one of the final steps in mitosis is the incorporation of a specific glycolipid into the plasma membrane, this event may represent a switch point for the entry of the cell into a new round of division (G_1) or the resting state (G_0). Activation of this switch may in turn be influenced by membrane-mediated information from outside the cell. Transformed cells may always be synthesizing and "on" switch or may not be able to synthesize an "off" switch such as the inability to synthesize the more complex gangliosides. Until we know more about the function and regulation of these sialic acid containing compounds, we can only speculate upon these possibilities.

REFERENCES

(1) P. T. Mora, R. O. Brady, R. M. Bradley and V. W. McFarland, Proc. Nat. Acad. Sci. USA, 63 (1969) 1290.

(2) R. O. Brady, C. Borek and R. M. Bradley, J. Biol. Chem., 244 (1969) 6552.

(3) I. Dijong, P. T. Mora and R. O. Brady, Biochemistry, 10 (1971) 4039.

(4) P. H. Fishman, V. W. McFarland, P. T. Mora and R. O. Brady, Biochem. Biophys. Res. Commun., 48 (1972) 48.

(5) F. A. Cumar, R. O. Brady, E. H. Kolodny, V. W. McFarland and P. T. Mora, Proc. Nat. Acad. Sci. USA, 67 (1970) 575.

(6) P. H. Fishman, R. O. Brady, R. M. Bradley, S. A. Aaronson and G. J. Todaro, Proc. Nat. Acad. Sci. USA, 71 (1974) in press.

(7) R. O. Brady and P. T. Mora, Biochim. Biophys. Acta, 218 (1970) 308.

(8) P. T. Mora, P. H. Fishman, R. H. Bassin, R. O. Brady and V. W. McFarland, Nature 245 (1973) 226.

(9) J. F. Tallman and R. O. Brady, Biochim. Biophys Acta, 293 (1973) 434.

(10) W. Eckhart, Nature 224 (1969) 1069.

(11) P. T. Mora, F. A. Cumar and R. O. Brady, Virology, 46 (1971) 60.

(12) R. E. Pollack, H. Green and G. J. Todaro, Proc. Nat. Acad. Sci. USA, 60 (1968) 126.

(13) R. E. Pollack, S. Wolman and A. Vogel, Nature, 228 (1970) 938.

(14) P. H. Fishman, R. O. Brady and P. T. Mora, in: Tumor Lipids: Biochemistry and Metabolism, ed. R. Wood (Am. Oil. Chem. Soc., Champaign, Ill., 1973) p. 251.

(15) R. O. Brady, P. H. Fishman and P. T. Mora, Federation Proc., 32 (1973) 102.

(16) R. O. Brady, P. H. Fishman and P. T. Mora, in: Advances in Enzyme Regulation, Vol. 11, ed. G. Weber (Pergamon, Oxford, 1973) p. 231.

(17) D. R. Dubbs, S. Kitt, R. A. deTorres and M. Anken, J. Virology, 1 (1967) 968.

(18) H. C. Renger and C. Basilico, Proc. Nat. Acad. Sci. USA, 69 (1972) 109.

(19) R. Sheinin, K. Onodera, G. Yogeeswaran and R. K Murray, in: The Biology of Oncogenic Viruses, IInd LePetit Symposium, ed. L. G. Silvestri (North Holland, Amsterdam, 1971) p. 274.

(20) V. N. Nigam, R. Lallier and C. Brailovsky, J. Cell. Biol., 58 (1973) 307.

(21) C. N. Wiblin and I. Macpherson, Int. J. Cancer, 12 (1973) 148.

(22) G. Yogeeswaran, R. Sheinin, J. R. Wherrett and R. K Murray, J. Biol. Chem., 247 (1972) 5146.

(23) H. Diringer, G. Strobel and M. A. Koch, Hoppe-Seyler's Z. physiol. Chem., 353 (1972) 1769.

(24) R. H. Bassin, L. A. Phillips, M. J. Kramer, D. K Haapala, P. T. Peebles, S. Nomura and P. J. Fischinger, Proc. Nat. Acad. Sci. USA, 68 (1971) 1520.

(25) S. A. Aaronson and W. P. Rowe, Virology, 42 (1970) 9.

(26) P. H. Fishman, S. A. Aaronson and R. O. Brady, unpublished observations.

(27) K. Hirai and V. Defendi, J. Virology, 9 (1972) 705.

(28) L. A. Babiuk and J. B. Hudson, Biochem. Biophys. Res. Commun., 47 (1972) 111.

(29) G. Marin and J. W. Littlefield, J. Virology, 2 (1968) 69.

(30) M. Weiss, B. Ephrussi and L. Scaletta, Proc. Nat. Acad. Sci. USA, 59 (1958) 1132.

(31) M. M. Burger, Federation Proc. 32 (1973) 91.

(32) S. J. Singer and G. L. Nicholson, Science,175 (1972) 720.

(33) S. Roseman, Chem. Phys. Lipids, 5 (1970) 270.

(34) R. J. Winzler, in: Int. Rev. Cytol., Vol. 29, eds. G. H. Bourne and J. F. Danielli (Academic Press, New York, 1970) p. 77.

(35) H.-D. Klenk and P. W. Choppin, Proc. Nat. Acad. Sci. USA, 66 (1970) 57.

(36) O. Renkonen, C. G. Gahmberg, K. Simons and L. Kaariainen, Acta Chem. Scand., 24 (1970) 733.

(37) P. Cuatrecasas, Biochemistry, 12 (1973) 3558.

(38) P. H. Fishman, M. D. Hollenberg and P. Cuatrecasas, unpublished observations

(39) H. S. Smith, G. D. Sher and G. J. Todaro, Virology, 44 (1971) 359.

(40) H. B. Bosmann and R. A. Winston, J. Cell. Biol., 45 (1970) 23.

(41) S. Chatterjee, C. C. Sweeley and L. F. Velicer, Biochem. Biophys. Res. Commun., 54 (1973) 585.

DISCUSSION

I. MacPherson, Imperial Cancer Research Fund Laboratories: Do you know if any of the glycolipids in the NRK line are density dependent?

P.H. Fishman, National Institutes of Health: In the NRK, yes, ceramidetrihexoside, a neutral glycolipid, for which I think Dr. McPherson has presented the structure, appears to be density dependent as there is an increase in this glycolipid when the normal cells increase in density.

S. Chatterjee, Michigan State University: Rosenberg, who has also worked on normal and virus-transformed cells tells us that there is a relationship between increased ganglioside catabolism and increased malignancy whereas your data shows a decrease in sugar transferase activity. Would you like to comment on that?

P.H. Fishman: I can only comment on our work. Originally when we observed these changes in gangliosides, we said well maybe it is a clue to increased catabolism. So we examined the sialidase activity, that is the enzyme that removes the sialic acid from GM_3 and GD_{1a}. There was no increase or decrease in sialidase activity when we compared virus-transformed mouse cells to normal mouse cells. I can't comment on Dr. Rosenberg's studies.

S. Chatterjee: I have one more question. In some of your studies you showed there was a decrease in the GD_{1a} level of about 80%. Do you notice the precursor of GD_{1a} on your thin-layer plates?

P.H. Fishman: You mean whether the GM_1, which is the precursor of GD_{1a} increases?

S. Chatterjee: Yes.

P.H. Fishman: Well, the glycosyltransferase block that we observed in that particular case (Moloney sarcoma virus-transformed cells) was the amino sugar transferase that converts GM_3 to GM_2 so therefore we were missing all of the higher homologs that is GM_2, GM_1, and GD_{1a}. So if anything would accumulate, it would be this component (GM_3). In some instances we do see an increase in that component.

S. Chatterjee: But your GM_3 levels didn't show a change?

P.H. Fishman: No. I have no explanation for that.

S. Steiner, Baylor College of Medicine: In the NRK system you focused on the hematoside but from the thin-layer figure, there are apparently are apparently were less mobile gangliosides. What was the status of these components?

P.H. Fishman: There were not any less mobile gangliosides. The less mobile components which migrate similarly to GD_{1a} are not gangliosides. We detect the gangliosides by spraying the thin-layer chromatogram with resorcinol reagent and then heating it. This reagent gives a specific blue color for sialic acid-containing compounds. The material you are refering to produces a yellow-brown color.

S. Steiner: I see, so the hematoside is it?

P.H. Fishman: Yes, this seems to be a problem because from what I understand Dr. David Critchley in Dr. MacPherson's lab has looked at NRK and in the cell line that they're using, there seems to be some higher ganglioside components. But the cell lines that we get from Dr. Aaronson do not have any higher gangliosides. They only have the GM_3. So it may be the way in which the cells are initially selected. These are new-born rat kidneys that are minced up, put in culture, and then you establish a cell line from such a preparation. You may get different cell types coming out depending on how you select them. I should say, in almost all cases, we are working with cloned cell lines and not just primary or secondary cell lines.

J. Schultz, Papanicolaou Cancer Research Institute: First, I want to congratulate Dr. Brady and Dr. Fishman who are associates on a beautiful piece of work and those who didn't stay to hear it certainly missed an awful lot. The question I want to ask is, during the period of time Dr. Brady worked in this area, are there any other ganglioside metabolism deficiences, not associated with cancer that you can tell us about? Is this something highly characteristic and specific for cancer, or are there other deficiencies that are related to it?

P.H. Fishman: Well, the only deficiencies that I can think of are well established. There is of course all the great work that Dr. Roscoe Brady has done on the lipid storage diseases specifically the glycosphingo-lipid storage diseases, such as Tay Sachs disease, and here we have the reverse situation, in that we have an accumulation of a ganglioside due to a defect in catabolism, that is the hexosaminidase that is involved in the breakdown of GM_2 is deficient in people with Tay Sachs disease, and they end up accumulating large amounts of GM_2 which results in severe neurological disorders and it's a very, very serious disease. So it's kind of the reverse of what we're seeing in viral transformation. It's a block in catabolism whereas with malignant transformation there is a block in biosynthesis of glycolipids.

A 4
B 5
C 6
D 7
E 8
F 9
G 0
H 1
I 2
J 3